Ilhenaylh

FEAST

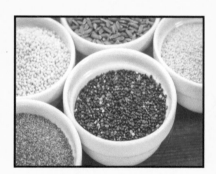
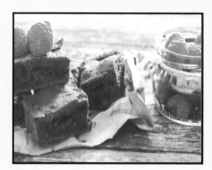
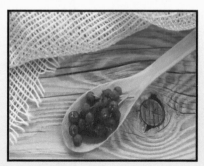
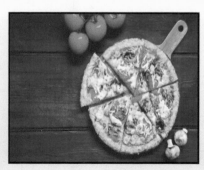

Ilhenaylh

FEAST

YVONNE WYSS

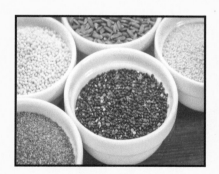
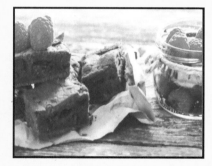
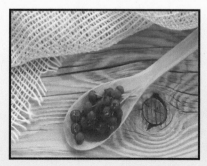
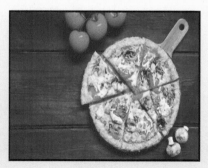

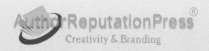
AuthorReputationPress®
Creativity & Branding

Author Reputation Press LLC
45 Dan Road Suite 5
Canton MA 02021
www.authorreputationpress.com
Hotline: 1(888) 821-0229
Fax: 1(508) 545-7580

Ordering Information:
Quantity sales. Special discounts are available on quantity purchases by corporations, associations, and others. For details, contact the publisher at the address above.

Printed in the United States of America.
ISBN-13:   Softcover   978-1-64961-772-9
                eBook   978-1-64961-773-6

Library of Congress Control Number: 2021917524

Here is the second edition to our first book. The re-do is to share our families journey and helpful information on gluten-free foods, recipes, and cooking that has worked for our family. It is not meant to be used, nor should it be used, to diagnose or treat any medical condition. For diagnosis or treatment of any medical problem, consult your own physician. The publisher and author are not responsible for any specific health or allergy needs that may require medical supervision and are not liable for any damages or negative consequences resulting from any treatment, action, application, or preparation to any person reading or following the information in this book. References are provided for informational purposes only and do not constitute endorsement of any websites or other sources. Readers should be aware that the websites listed in this book may change.

Education is the key in the world of gluten free! Read your labels and understand what you are buying. Fewer ingredients are always the best option. The less processing, the better. If you are not sure what an ingredient is, then research until you gain a better understanding of it. And keep in mind that natural does not always equal good for you!

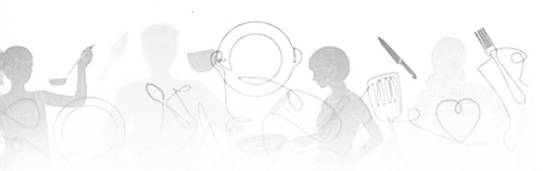

DEDICATION

This book is dedicated to those special people who have journeyed with me throughout my life, shaping my passion for food, cooking, and gluten-free healthy living.

My Partner Ken Drury – You have inspired me to stretch my horizons on food and have renewed my outlook on how we fuel and look after the machines we call our bodies. Thank you for eating all my burnt offerings and appreciating and trying everything with enthusiasm and kindness. You are my hero.

My children Tasha, Nicklaus, Brandon, and Tyler, and Riel – all the trials and your honesty makes it worth it. Thank you all for your honest opinions about what is good and what sucks!

My mother – I remember being a little girl and asking you to teach me to bake pies like Granny. I harassed you until you taught me how to make pastry dough. You were stunned— you couldn't bake a pie; you could explain the process perfectly! Thank you for being an amazing teacher.

My father – When I was a child, you were the chief cook in our family. Using your expertise as a meatcutter, you taught me how to clean and can fish, and how to cut and process all meat. You showed me how to preserve vegetables and fruit. You brought your Swiss influence and your passion for hunting and fishing to our life, as well as an appreciation of our country and its wildlife. My own love of the outdoors reflects your bright influence, and with gratitude, I raise my hands to you now. Thank you for passing on such wonderful teachings.

My granny – My earliest memories are of you taking your pies to Mosquito Creek Marina to sell. What an incredible matriarch, finding ways to feed your large family of nine children. She was also known as a master cedar basket weaver and matriarch of our family

My other mom Nancy – You guided and inspired my cooking and baking skills, and I love sharing recipes with you. Thank you for teaching me to appreciate all cultures and their food. Thank you for helping me see food as medicine and how central it was to a home – even frying an onion gave the hints of food to come...

My uncle Maurice – You shared with me how and why the concept of ilhenaylh is important to our people, and your teachings are invaluable. Huychewx! Hiy Hiy! Miigwetch! Thank you!

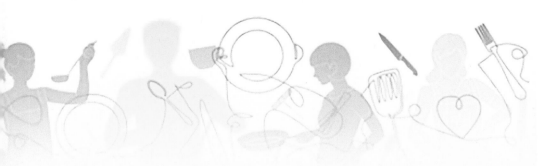

Origins

Health and wellness include the physical, mental, spiritual, emotional cultural, environmental, social, and economic well-being of you, your family, your community, your nation . . . and all your relations!

—Elder's wisdom, *Berry Cakes*

Ilhenaylh (ill-hen-ail) means "feast" in the Squamish language. As an Aboriginal Matriarch of Khahtsahlano (Squamish) and Sto:lo First peoples of British Columbia on the West Coast of Canada, Our Family is the lineage of the first family of Haat'sa'lanexw from Chaythoos and XwayXway. I offer a journey into some of my families traditional approaches to food. Much of our learning was through oral transmission – teachings that have continued to guided my life. I share some of these teachings throughout my book.

The custom of My people was to always cook extra food for guests. This tradition is similar to other Indigenous cultures as my partner who is Cree Metis from Manito-api, otherwise know as Manitoba, confers the same teaching that was customary in his community and people. Most of Indigenous families did not have much, but what they had they were always willing to share. It was viewed by our communities that our family and friends gave of their time to be with us which was seen as an honor, so we honored them by sharing a meal with them, as we do not know when they ate last. This goes back to a time when people would travel great distances by canoe or on foot to attend ceremonial gatherings or celebrations. Food would always be ready for them to take back on their journey home. Generosity and hospitality continue to be among the greatest values held by the Khahtsahlano people.

The Khahtsahlano believe it is important to prepare oneself in a good way when planning to invite people to share a meal and their time. Being in a positive frame of mind is essential when preparing and cooking food, because, in turn, the food is infused with all these positive and heartfelt thoughts. This acts as a blessing for guests.

Indigenous philosophy teaches that health equals not only freedom from disease, but also a robust body, mind, and spirit. Thus, through experience and the teachings of their elders, succeeding Indigenous generations have learned to select foods in proper amounts to supply the body with the required nutrients. Food is not only a source of energy and vitality, but also medicine.

Historically speaking, plant and animal life were considered sacred by the Khahtsahlano and therefore never to be wasted or taken unnecessarily. There was a strongly held belief that the animals and plants entered into a contract with the Creator to offer themselve as a way to care for us humans, and without these relationships, we would be helpless in this world. This is why our people believe it important to have good kinship relations with all of creation. this relationship was often expressed through legends and daily customs. Thus, this cookbook contains teachings and anecdotes pertaining to the legends and daily food customs cultivated over tens of thousands of years by Khahtsahlano people. These can be stories or snippets of indigenous wisdom geared toward offering cultural perspective and encouraging overall balance in lifestyle and health.

By highlighting dietary changes that have arisen from the consumption of traditional to more modern foods, this book seeks ways to blend both categories through gluten-free cooking, something that is especially close to my heart. Gluten Free is a new term, one that was not part of our traditional foods, and our journey was learning process to uncover our the history and journey to bring our family closer to tradional foods and healthy eating for our family.

How It All Began . . . The Journey to Traditional Living

I write this book with the hope of leaving an impression on people why it is important to change how we look at food. Gluten free living is not about cutting things out – it is about changing the way you eat and look at food. This book is written from my world view as an Indigenous Matriarch living in Canada and all the experiences it includes. I live within the Lower Mainland of British Columbia lies the Traditional territory of Xwemelch'stn (Homulcheson) – known today by the colonial name of Skwxwu7mesh Uxumixw (Squamish Nation). I would like to share some of my culture through food.

Our path to gluten-free living is different and required learning a new way of embracing food, but it doesn't have to be hard. It seems that as awareness of the effects of gluten has increased in recent years, more and more people are taking a closer look at just how gluten might be affecting their lives and the lives of their loved ones. During my own journey, as I educated myself on gluten, I discovered that this protein derived from wheat and related grains can be found in many food products, and sometimes even in those one would never expect to find it in. Many people's bodies cannot adequately process this protein, which explains why it leads to a variety of digestive and other health-related problems.

There is a notable distinction between the separate categories of people who cannot digest gluten. There are people with celiac disease, for example, in which the lining of the intestine becomes damaged due to exposure to gluten. There are those with gluten intolerance. Allergies and intolerance are different. I am intolerant, whereas my partner and his son are allergic. What does this mean? It means that they will have allergic reactions, while I will experience discomfort, like inflammation in joints and muscles. Either way, by eliminating or minimizing gluten from our diets as much as possible, we can hope to avoid adverse health effects and enjoy better quality of life.

I wrote this book to share our food journey and we discovered that many foods we cosume today are not easily digested in most indigneous preople, which is evidenced in the higher rates of obsetity, heart disease, and diabetes. As Indigenous people, our diets have relevatively changed dramatically since the industrialization of food in the mid 20th century, and much research today suggests that this rapid change has created metabolic imbalances for some by way of their ability to motabilize the proteins in grains that contain gluten, but more importantly, in foods that are highly processed. Gluten-free living is not about cutting things out; it is about changing the way one eats and looks at food. Please note that this book has been influenced by experiences that are specific to those within my home, and the recipes that I created is what has been successful for my family. Use the recipes as a guide to explore your own processes for cooking and find ways to learn how to eat well for your family.

I hope that you enjoy this book, and it assists you in making choices that work for your family. May your food journey guide you as it did ours and provide you and your family with the positive and enjoyable experiences as it did for mine.

Huychewx! Hiy Hiy! Ninanaskomowin Miyosin Pimatisowin -Gratitude for a beautiful life.

Yvonne

CONTENTS

SAVORY

SWEET

PLANTS AND HERBS

Measures

lb = pound	L = litre	T = tablespoon
kg = kilogram	C = cup	t = teaspoon
Q = quart	Oz = ounce	g = gram

Adjustments for Recipes in Other Provinces

Please note that the liquid measures and cooking temperatures listed for my recipes are based on my location in British Columbia. It is important to remember that if you live in another province, you must make the appropriate adjustments to achieve the best results. As a veteran cook and baker, I can tell you that this is necessary because altitude and air pressure affect recipes. For example, if you are located in Manitoba, you will need to add almost an additional three-fourths to a full cup of water to your pancake batter in order to get the same consistency. Allow for more baking time as well for cakes and other similar items, and make sure to do your toothpick tests prior to removing your baked goods from the oven so that they are properly cooked through.

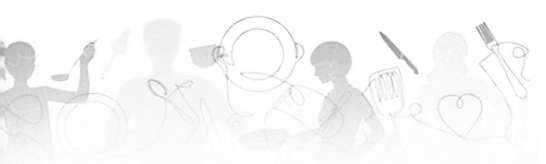

Gluten-Free Flours

Almond

Almond meal is a very expensive but great option for baking. It adds wonderful flavour and texture. I use this extensively in crumbles, bars, squares, tarts, and crusts for pies. It makes wonderful keto biscuits as well.

Coconut

Coconut flour is used for baking and has a terrific smell, but it is very spongy and requires a lot of liquid to work with, up to 3x's the liquid in recipes to ensure moisture in the finished product. It is not well suited for binding, though it has a great flavour and is good in small amounts for blending. Though it is not my preference to use coconut flour in my baking, I do use other forms of coconut, such as oil, nectar, and sugar. These are all wonderful products that are low in glycemic value and high in fibre, nutrients, and other vitamins. The XO Baking Company uses coconut flour in their blend and the boxed cake mixes are fantastic and make wonderful quick gluten free desserts that are crowd pleasing.

Corn

This is not the best alternative in my home because of its generally high level of processing and additives. I might use corn chips, for example, but not cornstarch. I use tapioca instead, as it is less likely to cause allergic reactions in my family members. I have used corn flour, but only in limited quantities.

GMO is a term tossed around today and not necessarily defined. This abbreviation stands for "genetically modified organism." The majority of corn today is genetically modified unless otherwise specified as being organic, and the latter is not always readily available. Corn is a crop that is used in everything from fuel to medication. A source of controversy, it is nevertheless cheap to produce, is versatile, and is thus heavily funded by the government and supported by big companies. Through my research, I have found that corn is not as gluten free or as safe for those with gluten intolerance as we are led to believe, either. One has to be careful in seeking out information about what is safe to use.

Fava Bean, Other Beans

Bean flours are widely used in gluten-free cooking. They are good sources of protein, even in small amounts, as well as stable additions to blends. Some have an aftertaste. Many commercial blends of flours have some type of bean flour in their blends. They are reasonably priced and readily available but may not be the best option for people with gas and intestinal issues.

Quinoa

This is a complete protein. It has an even flavour that is slightly nutty. In small quantities in a blend, it provides stability and protein needed for nutrition. It's great for breads and biscuits. Small amounts are good for using in bars and squares. I use quinoa in the following forms: flakes, seeds, and flour. I use it as a complete protein for cooking and baking, adding it to puddings, stir-fry dishes, and flours. This ancient grain is an all-around source of nutrition that gets a lot of regular use in my home.

Rice

Wild rice, sweet rice, brown rice—there are many. Be mindful of your choices, though, as some have flavours that you may not want in your baking.

Wild Rice – This sustainable food source is the perfect food with 11% plant protein and used in so many ways for traditional dishes to gravies and soups. The flour for this is very rice and dense in colour and flavour. Does not bind well but adds wonderful flavor to soups and gravies.

Potato Starch

This starch is extracted from the cell roots of potato tubers of the plant. The use of this starch is compatible with tapioca and Corn in baking and cooking purposes. This forms part of the blend of flour used in many of the recipes here in this book.

Sorghum

Also known as *Sorghum bicolor*, this is a species of grass. It is grown mainly in Africa, Central America, and South Asia. Cultivated for its grain, which is widely used in poor and rural villages, it is a major world crop that is also utilized for making "syrup," molasses, and alcoholic beverages. Sorghum is considered one of the five most important food crops in the world. I use it in flour form in my own flour blends.

Tapioca

This is used as a starch. In the starch form, it adds no flavour for use in cooking gravies, bars, squares—just about everything. I use it as a staple in all my cooking. As a granulated crystal, it is perfect for making fruit jams, pies, and compotes. Tapioca thickens, but does not affect colour or clarity in fruit, nor does it add any flavour.

Teff

This is one of the smallest ancient grains. From a grass family similar to sorghum, teff grows on long stems also referred to as lovegrass. It is native to northeast Africa and southwestern Arabia and has long been widely used in Ethiopia. The seeds are so tiny that they are easily lost, and the word "teff" itself means "lost" in the Amharic language.

Teff flour is a dark, heavy flour I mix in small quantities into my flour blends. It adds a high fibre content. In addition, this small grain gives the body three main types of energy: fast release, slow release, and endurance. Its nutritional value is phenomenal. It aids in muscle building and tissue repair, and provides calcium, magnesium, and vital minerals and vitamins for growth.

Millet

A mild flavoured grain that when toasted has a nutty almost corn flavour. The flour is yellow, consistency of fine powder. The blends well with starches and rice flour to make a light baking four for cookies, cakes, muffins and scones. Its mild flavour doesn't overpower fine baking and vanilla. I like this for my finer flour to use in brownies, muffins, cookies and pies. The cakes with this flour in the blend are fluffier.

Teaching

In my personal journey and experimentations, I have found that the best way to be confident with gluten-free flours is to take a recipe you are really familiar with and adjust it with a gluten-free substitute until you are happy with the results. By using your own recipe, you can make adjustments until it works to your liking. It is like chemistry—try and try again until you succeed!

I spent ten years creating flour blends that has the closest consistency to the gluten alternative and is perfect for all-purpose substitution in all recipes. These blends offer a more neutral taste that does not overpower cakes, shortbread cookies, or any other delicate desserts. It rises well in yeast breads and in regular baking. It is also a terrific alternative to thickeners for making gravy and sauces. I use a couple of flour blends throughout, one is heavier for more grain-based breads, and buns. The other flour blend is lighter and less strongly flavored grains to use for finer baking like cookies, cakes and pies.

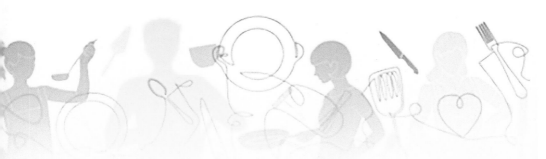

THICKENERS, BINDERS, OILS, SUBSTITUTIONS, AND OTHER ADDITIONS

Guar Gum

A type of polysaccharide, guar gum is the ground endosperm of guar beans. It allows binding, is a powerful thickening agent, and has almost eight times the elasticity of cornstarch. The only downside I see for this product is that it falls under the classification of a bean. So, if you have difficulties with bean-based items, you might want to stick with xanthan gum.

Xanthan Gum

This gum is a polysaccharide, a carbohydrate secreted by the bacterium *Xanthomonas campestris*. It was discovered by Allene Rosalind Jeanes and her research team at the United States Department of Agriculture in the 1950s and has been widely used since the 1960s in the food industry as a food-thickening agent. Check ingredient lists on products at the grocery store just for fun and see if you can find it!

A Note on Gums: I sometimes combine guar gum and xanthan gum. When used together, their elasticity and binding potency create a result that is the closest to gluten but without its potential negative effects. Though each can be used on its own, combined they create a more stable product that is better for baking and consistency. In this case I use equal parts xanthan and guar gums.

If you have four cups total of gluten-free flours, then add one teaspoon of either combined gums or just the one you prefer for every cup of flour. But keep in mind that some recipes ask for less of the gums. This is why I tend to add gums later when I am baking and to blend my flours without the gums, as I am never sure of what gum levels are required for a specific recipe. Pizza utilizes a higher gum content due to the need for dough elasticity, for example. Conversely, biscuits need less gum to bind them and keep them fluffy and airy. Bars and squares need little or no gum at all to make them crumbly and melty. Choose and apply your gum combination when you bake rather than putting it into your blend first.

Buttermilk

To make my version of buttermilk, add one teaspoon of lemon juice to one cup of soy, coconut, or almond milk and let stand for a couple of minutes. Traditional buttermilk is a soured milk culture, and lemon juice creates the chemical reaction needed for this. I use alternatives to cow's milk due to the lactose issues in my home. My kids don't notice a difference in any dishes I prepare with this buttermilk recipe, so I think it is quite comparable to traditional buttermilk.

Gluten

This is a composite protein that for some people does not break down in the body and that subsequently causes problems in those with gluten intolerance. Because it is not properly processed, gluten builds up in the body and causes things like "leaky gut." It is a binding agent that provides the lovely, fluffy stickiness found in regular flour and flour-based foods. All but one recipe in this book completely exclude gluten.

Coconut Oil

A personal favorite in my home, this versatile oil contains lauric acid (a saturated fat found in breast milk) and has many health benefits, such as lowering HDL cholesterol in the blood, making it a good option for diabetics. It can restore normal thyroid function, which is important for overall body function. And it helps fight off viral and bacterial infections, and fungal infections, including those caused by candida. By adding this wonder oil to your normal diet, you can significantly boost your immune system.

Olive Oil

Many properties in olive oil are believed to promote good health. Oleocanthal, a phytonutrient, is said to mimic ibuprofen and assist in reducing inflammation. Squalene, which aids in biosynthesis, and lignans, a class of antioxidants, are other positive attributes of olive oil. It is low in saturated fat, high in antioxidants, and contains carotenoids, which are good for protecting against UV rays. I use extra virgin cold pressed, the oil that is extracted during the first pressing and is of the highest and purest quality.

Walnut Oil

Though it is starting to become more popular, this oil is expensive and hard to obtain. I found it first in a natural food store and then of all places at Liquidation World. I use it sparingly and usually only for salads and wild rice pastas once they are at the serving stage. This oil is tasty and offers excellent nutritional value. A real treat!

Earth Balance Butter, Earth Balance Shortening

Both of these products are excellent. I use only the sticks, and not the spread, though this brand makes a coconut spread that is wonderful and amazing! I like to use the shortening sticks for pastries and bannock—it's great for baking. The butter sticks work just as well. You don't need a lot, and these products are good especially if you have family members with vegan preferences, or reactions to other fats and trouble with dairy.

Dough Improver

Here is a simple recipe for a stabilizing gluten-free baking agent:

2 C (500 ml) granulated soy lecithin or rice lecithin
1 T ascorbic acid
1 T ground ginger
Grind the soy or rice lecithin in a food processor or blender until a powdery consistency is achieved. The texture of lecithin is sticky and dry; it feels tacky to the touch. Mix in the ginger and ascorbic acid and store in a dry container. It will keep for months. to stabilize baking use one to one and a half teaspoons are usually required per recipe.

Vinegar

It is amazing how many different uses this acid has. It is utilized for preserving and creating everything from sauces to salsa. Vinegar has been a no-go in my home because it facilitates yeast growth, so I had to find an alternative: lime juice or lemon juice.

Apple Cider Vinegar

A natural vinegar which contains a mother through the fermenting process. This vinegar is perfect for using within the bread process, and any substitute for acids in baking.

Other benefits of this vinegar when added with other things like honey, cayenne, turmeric, pepper as a tonic.

Sugars
There are so many varieties of sugars. They come in both natural and processed forms. There are up to thirty-seven varieties of sugar produced in the world today across seven different countries. Each has a different glycemic value.

Cane sugar is sucrose extracted from sugarcane and makes up 70 percent of the world's sugar. Brazil is one of the largest producers of sugarcane in the world. The remaining mass-scale sugar production comes from beet sugar, which is also used for commercial purposes.

Honey is another popularly used sweetener. Honey offers properties of local life bees visit through their harvesting of pollen. Pollen in honey offers immune strengthening properties. When used in moderation, it can help fight off colds and the flu. An ounce of prevention!

Honey unpasteurized should not be fed to infants, as it can be toxic to their intestinal tracts. So be sure to do your research when deciding what types of sweeteners to use when baking and cooking. Sugars have glycemic values, which affects how they are digested and how the body creates insulin, especially in the case of diabetics. For example, processed cane sugar has a glycemic value between eighty and one hundred. Honey has a glycemic value of thirty-one to seventy-eight, depending upon the processing of the honey.

Coconut sugar has a glycemic value of thirty. This sugar comes in a powder form as well as a nectar which is like a syrup. The sugar is refined from the plant and the flowers. This sugar is one used in several recipes here. The sugar is very rich and almost molasses like in colour and texture when used in cooking.

The use of alternative lower glycemic sugars in many of the recipes I use in this book can impact the impact of sugar digestion for those who need to measure glycemic values. The recipes have all been adjusted to accommodate alternative sugars.

Spices

Herbamare is a spice mixture by Alfred Vogel, a renowned Swiss naturopath. Made with sea salt, celery, leeks, cress, onions, chives, parsley, lovage, garlic, marjoram, rosemary, thyme, and kelp, and free of MSG, gluten, lactose, milk protein, additives, and preservatives, it is an excellent natural product that can be picked up at local grocery stores. This spice mix can be used with most savory dishes. I use it in many of my recipes. I cook for my elderly parents a lot, and this suits them fine. It is often the only spice I can get my father, who has dementia, to eat.

Turmeric and Pepper – combined these are well known for their anti-inflammatory properties. I use this combination in the spicing of Wild rice stir fry and accompanying stews, soups and roasts.

Vanilla Bean, Extract and Powder: The extract comes in many formats such as pure extract, organic which does not use sugar but uses alcohol and imitation which has additives. The bean can be used and scraped to take the vanilla out and then the outer hull can be put in anything you cook to extract the most use of your vanilla bean flavor. The powder form of Vanilla bean is the most versatile. Dried ground vanilla bean and can be added to all recipes.

Gluten-Free Flour Blends
I have created two gluten-free flour blends that are "all purpose" flours. These blends are versatile and work for all recipes in the book, including those with and without yeast.

Signature Blend – lighter baking

1 C tapioca flour	1 C rice flour
1 C potato starch	1 C Millet flour

Blend and store mixture in a large Tupperware container. Use as needed. This blend is lighter and has less strong flavor for cakes, muffins, scones and cookies.

These items can be purchased at local grocery stores such as Bulk

House Blend

1 Cup sorghum flour	¼ Cup quinoa flour
1 Cup tapioca starch	¼ Cup teff flour

Mix all ingredients together and put in a container for storage in the fridge or freezer. It is a good idea to prepare small batches, as gluten-free flours tend to have shorter shelf lives than regular all-purpose flours. Yields vary.

Historical Points of Interest

My great grandfather six generations back Chief August Jack was well known in the late 1930s as a storyteller and was recorded by Major J. S. Matthews, a city archivist of Vancouver. The following is an excerpt about early Squamish life:

"Whiteman's food change everything," said August Khatsahlano in a conversation while we sat at lunch in a downtown restaurant. "Indians had plenty of food long ago, but I could not do without tea and sugar now. These days Indians who do not want tea and sugar know nothing about it. Lots of meat, bear, deer, beaver, cut up meat in strips and dry—no part wasted, not even guts—fill him up with something good, make sausage, just like Whiteman's. Only head wasted; throw head away. Then salmon—plenty salmon. Sturgeon, flounder, trout, lots all sorts of fish; come sun-dried; lots crab and clam on beach.

"But Whiteman's food change everything. Everywhere Whiteman goes he change food. China, other places, he always changes food where he goes.

"I was born Snauq, the old Indian village under the Burrard Bridge. When I little boy I listen to old people talk. Old people say Indians' first Whiteman's near Squamish. When they first see ship, they think it an island with three dead trees, might be schooner, might be sloop; two mast and bowsprit, sails tied up. Indian Braves in about twenty canoes come down Squamish River, go see. Get nearer, canoes come down Squamish River, go see. Get nearer, see men on island; men have black clothes with high hat coming to point at top. Think most likely black uniform and great coat turned up collar like priest cowl.

"Whiteman's give Indians ship's biscuits; Indian not know what

biscuit for. Before Whiteman come Indian have little balls, not very big, roll them along ground, shoot them with bow and arrow for practice, teach young Indian so as not to miss deer. Just the same you use clay pigeon. Indian not know ship's biscuits good to eat, so roll them along ground like little practice balls, shoot at them, break them up."

Savory

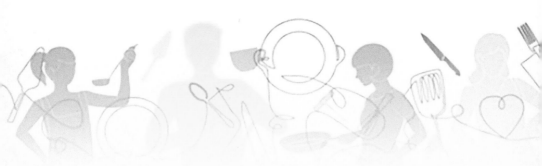

DEER ROAST WITH MOCK MASHED POTATOES

Deer Roast:

4 shallots quartered
4 lb deer roast
2 t Herbamare seasoning (or your choice of seasoning)
¼ C fat
olive oil
pepper to taste
salt to taste

Mock Mashed Potatoes:

1 head cauliflower
1 C ricotta cheese
salt to taste
pinch of nutmeg

Boil the cauliflower until it is soft in a large dutch oven pot. Once cooked until completely soft, drain in a colander and return to dutch oven to mash it. Add the ricotta cheese, salt, and nutmeg. Mix until everything is well blended. Use a stick blender if you want to further cream the cauliflower. This dish is low in fat and a nice meal replacement for potatoes.

Turn oven to 350 degrees. Put the deer roast in a roasting pan. I use a clay roasting pan, as this keeps the meat tender and retains heat for roasting. Put the crushed garlic, a bit of olive oil, and salt and pepper to taste on the deer roast. You can also add turmeric, rosemary, and sage. Roast for about three hours. This will cook a 4-pound roast.

Serve with my mock mashed potatoes or with regular potatoes mashed with soy milk, butter, nutmeg, and salt. You can soak your potatoes for 20 minutes in a saltwater brine prior to boiling them to remove some of the starch and reduce the carbohydrate content as well. Make sure you rinse the potatoes and replace the water with clean water prior to boiling. I add a pinch of salt when I replace the water prior to boiling. I do this with my fries. It makes them a lower-calorie potato option.

Preparation time: 25 minutes   Serving: 8 servings
Cooking time: 3.5 hours   Calories per serving: 344

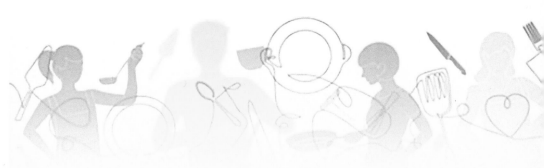

Bison Tourtière

Crust:

Use Pie Crust recipe (page 48) or purchase double crust premade shells)

Filling:

1lb ground bison
1 clove crushed garlic
½ cup olive oil
1 small-sized onion, finely chopped
1 C peas and carrots
1 t savory
¼ t ground cloves
¼ C tapioca starch
¼ C water

Preheat oven to 350 degrees.

Fry the onion and garlic in the olive oil. Add the ground bison and cook until browned. Add the spices, cloves, tapioca starch, water, and peas and carrots.

Roll out the pie crust and put it in a pie plate. Fill the pie crust with the cooked meat mixture and put the top crust over it. When I roll out pastry, I put the ball of dough between two pieces of parchment paper in order to keep it from sticking to the counter and to make it easier to transfer the pastry to the pie plate.   Once it is rolled out take the top parchment paper off and place this side down into the pie plate and remove the second piece of parchment paper as you settle the pastry into the pie plate.   Place the pie plate in the oven and bake for 30 minutes, until the top crust has cooked.

Serve with broth as gravy and side vegetables or wild rice.

Preparation time: 35 minutes
Cooking time: 20 minutes for meat filling
Baking time: 30 to 45 minutes
Yield: One 9-inch pie
Serving size: 1 piece of a 9-inch pie
Calories per serving: 357

Story Time

Ken once told me a story about how his mom used to make tourtière and how much he missed this traditional dish. I had also grown up with it being served at Christmas. So, I went to work coming up with a gluten-free version. Trying my hand at modifying my regular pie crust, I was able to adjust my old recipe to create a flexible and flaky gluten-free option. The next step was to use meat we could eat. For years, I had made tourtière with pork, so for a change, I used ground bison and added fats through olive oil as well as the spices and ingredients I had used with pork. I also found I needed to use gravy instead of fat because pork has a lot of fat in it and bison is very lean. This was a great compromise. I now make enough gravy to pour over the tourtière once it is baked. This is a regular meal in our home nowadays.

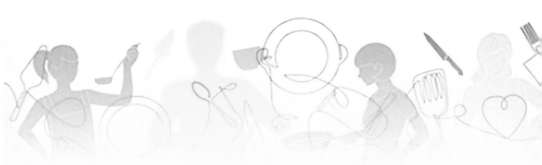

BISON SHEPHERD'S PIE

Filling:

2 C bison broth (see recipe under Broths)
2 T tapioca starch
1 lb. ground bison
1 clove crushed garlic
1 t olive oil
1 medium-sized onion, finely chopped
½ t Herbamare

1 C peas and carrots
pepper to taste - a pinch
salt to taste – a pinch

Topping:

1 head cauliflower
½ C ricotta cheese
½ t salt
Preheat oven to 350 degrees.

Sauté the onion, garlic, olive oil, Herbamare, salt, pepper, and bison together. Add the peas and carrots, tapioca, and broth. Heat until the tapioca is not cloudy and has thickened the broth.

Steam the head of cauliflower until it is soft. Mash it completely and remove all liquid by draining it thoroughly. Add the ricotta cheese and salt. Blend well. Use the same process as the Deer roast and mashed potatoes for cooking and mashing the cauliflower.

Put the meat mixture into a casserole dish. I like to use my stoneware casserole dish. The dimensions are approximately 8" x 4" x 4". Cover the meat mixture with the cauliflower topping.

Put the casserole dish in the oven and bake for 25 minutes. Then turn up the heat to 500 degrees and broil for another 5 minutes, until the cauliflower topping has browned slightly. You can add soy cheese on top if you want a slight variation of this dish.

Preparation time: 25 minutes
Cooking time: 20 minutes for cauliflower, shepherd's pie 30 minutes
Baking time: 30 minutes
Yield: 8 x 4 x 4 dish
Serving size: 1.5 cup serving for 6 servings
Calories per serving: 156

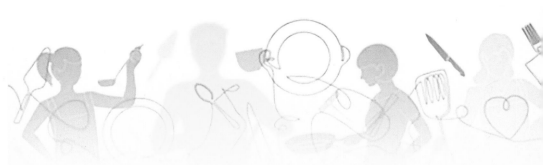

Bonnie's Chicken and Turkey Strips and Wings

2 kg chicken wings
2 kg boneless, skinless chicken thighs
2 C house blend
1 large boneless, skinless turkey thigh
2-4 T Olive oil
2 t MSG-free Hy's Seasoning Salt
a dash peppers

Note: I separate the turkey and the chicken onto different baking sheets because of allergy issues in my home. So, with that in mind, I also coat the turkey and chicken pieces in the flour.

Preheat oven to 375 degrees. Line two baking sheets with parchment paper. Put the wings on one of the baking sheets and sprinkle them with Himalayan Sea salt and pepper. Put them in the oven immediately, before you start the strips. They take longer to cook, about 45 minutes.

Cut the chicken and turkey into about ½-inch strips. Mix together the Hy's Seasoning Salt and the flour in a large Ziplock bag or a container with a lid that seals so you can shake the strips to coat them thoroughly. Take a handful of strips at a time and completely coat them in the flour and seasoning salt mix. Shake off the excess flour carefully and place the strips on the other parchment-lined baking sheet... Drizzle oil over all the strips Put the strips into the oven.

About 10 minutes into baking, flip the strips over and brown them on the other side. use thighs, as they already have some fat in them, and the meat is juicier than breast meat.

Fully cooked, the strips should be browned lightly on both sides and not overdone. They also travel very well as to-go snacks. I pack them for road trips and whenever my kids go to play sports.

Preparation time: 15 minutes
Baking time: 45 minutes for the wings
                20 minutes for the strips
Yield: 4.5 kg meat or approximately 9 lbs.
Serving size: ¾ lb. meat or .75kg per person or 10 servings
Calories per serving: 662

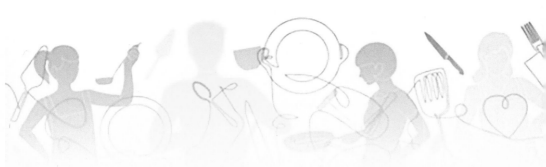

SALMON CAKES

2 T olive oil
2 cans salmon with bones and juice, crushed completely
2 T tapioca starch
1 T fresh or freeze-dried cilantro, finely chopped
1 T fresh or freeze-dried dill
1 egg white
½ C cooked quinoa
½ red or white onion, finely chopped
½ t turmeric
pepper to taste
salt to taste

Note: Used fresh, canned, or smoked, salmon was a very important food among First Nations peoples, especially the Khahtsahlano and Sto: lo—my people.

Mix all ingredients together and press into cakes. Add olive oil to a frying pan or a flat griddle and cook until the cakes are golden brown on each side.

It takes about half an hour from start to finish to make these easy, gluten-free, protein-packed salmon cakes. Salmon, of course, is high in omega-3 fatty acids and protein, and the quinoa adds another complete protein – try using the mixed red, black, and white quinoa together for texture and taste. Turmeric is a great spice that is high in antifungal properties.

Very nutritional and tasty, this is a great meal when you are in a hurry and need to feed the family fast.

Preparation time: 30 minutes
Cooking time: 10 minutes
Yield: 8 cakes
Serving size: 4 oz with 2 cakes per serving
Calories per serving: 226

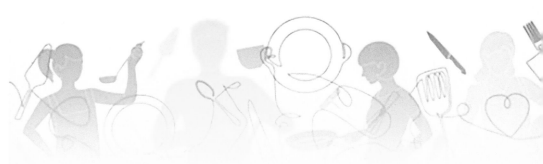

BARBECUED SALMON

cedar plank(s)
1 filleted side of salmon per plank (approximately 4 lbs.)

Place the salmon on the cedar plank(s). Grill the salmon until the white fat of the fish appears evenly over the surface of the fillet. This takes approximately 20 to 25 minutes, depending on the size of the fillet. A 4-pound fillet will take this amount of time. The key is to watch the salmon to ensure it has an even distribution of white. Leaving it to grill for any longer will dry out the salmon. In fact, it is better if the fillet is only partially white at its thickest point.

Cedar planks should be free of any chemical treatments or coatings. They are soaked in water for several hours prior to grilling to prevent burning. Submerging the planks in a baking pan of water works well. They must be weighted down to ensure they soak completely. Salmon fillets should be prepared so that they fit on the planks of cedar. Whole fillets can be placed on longer planks, while shorter ones can be used for salmon steaks. The salmon should be as fresh as possible. Wild salmon has the most flavor.

Preparation time: 10 minutes
Cooking time: 20 to 25 minutes
Yield: 4 - 1lb servings

Serving size: 1lb
Calories per serving: 85

Story Time

My grandfather taught my dad to cook fish our traditional way. We used the "ironwood" bush to cook salmon over an open fire. *Holodiscus discolor,* commonly known as ocean spray, creambush, or ironwood, is a shrub of western North America and is common in the Pacific Northwest, where it is found in both openings and the forest understory at low to moderate elevations.

When my dad came to Canada in the 1960s and met my mom, he was working for Canada Packers as a meatcutter, and my mom was working at the fish canneries near Terminal Avenue in Vancouver. My father loved the Native way of life and learned as many of the teachings as he could from my grandfather Lorne Whitton Nahanee and my grandmother Eva Mae Nahanee (Caufield). My grandfather used to get my dad to drive him to Squamish to harvest the ironwood for sticks to cook salmon on. My dad learned what trees to look for, and how to choose the straightest ones, clean them, and prepare them to cook fish on. My dad used to cook salmon this way. One of the biggest open pits was a 150-foot pit, cooking over 5,000 pieces of salmon for the Salmon Queen Festival in Steveston, British Columbia. He used mostly alder wood to cook with and would get the fires hot with a good base of coals. He would keep the fire stoked and put three pieces of spring salmon steak on each stick, cooking them until they were juicy and browned, dripping fat down the sticks. This is still my favorite way to eat salmon. It requires effort and work but is worth every morsel.

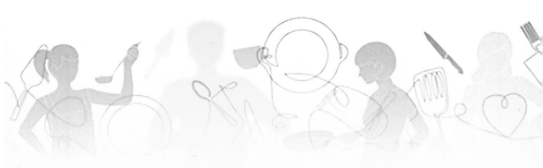

FISH AND CHIPS

Fish:

8 pieces sole, individually frozen
2 C gluten-free corn flakes (honey or plain)
¾ C soy, almond, or coconut milk
olive oil for frying

Chips:

4 large-sized potatoes
2 T olive oil
2 T salt + 2 T vinegar for soaking potatoes
1 T sea salt, paprika, or MSG-free Hy's Seasoning Salt
water to cover potatoes

Note: Gluten-free corn flakes can be purchased at Save-On-Foods, Superstores, natural foods stores, and most other grocery stores in the "Gluten-Free" section. I usually grind an entire large bag of corn flakes, then use a bit at a time in a bowl for dredging the fish. For the chips, you can use Idaho, white, or Yukon Gold potatoes. Choose whatever seasoning you prefer.

Preheat oven to 400 to 425 degrees.

Grind the corn flakes in a food processor. Then place 1 cup of ground corn flakes in a flat dish Put the soy, almond, or coconut milk in a bowl. Take one piece of fish and dip in the milk to soak before dredging it in the corn flakes. Then, fry the fish in olive oil for about 30 seconds per side, or until golden brown. You can judge based on what temperature you have set your stove burners. I usually estimate two pieces of fish per person,

For the chips, cut the potatoes into slices. Put them in a large bowl of water, add about 2 tablespoons of salt, and soak for about 20 minutes or more. This removes a lot of starch, which allows the chips to bake up crispier and makes them less heavy for those watching their diets. Remove the potato slices from the water, rinse, and pat dry. Coat them with olive oil and seasoning.

Line a large cookie sheet or jelly roll pan with parchment paper. Place the chips in the pan and bake for about 45 minutes. They will be crispy and yummy like the fried version, but healthier and without the calories! Make lots—they will not last!

Preparation time: 20 minutes
Cooking time: 1 minute per piece of sole
Baking time: 45 minutes for the chips

Yield: 4 servings
Serving size: 1 C chips and 2 pieces fish
Calories per serving: 599

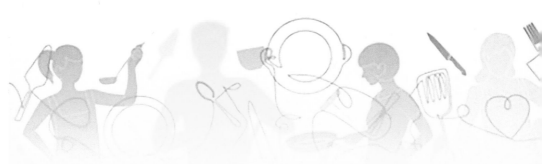

BONE BROTH

6 to 8 lbs. bones, knuckles or joints (3 kg)
4 bay leaves
2 T salt
2 T savory
1 clove garlic, with outer husk removed
1 large-sized onion, cut into quarters – or shallots
1 T pepper
fennel (or anise), cut into large pieces including Fronds
Herbamare
water to cover bones in pot (approximately 32 cups)

Note: I use the bones from any animals we have hunted or from meat obtained from the butcher. bison meat and large marrow bones make our favorite soup .

Preheat oven to 400 degrees. Take the bones and place them on a pan with the onions and garlic and roast in the oven for about 40 minutes. Take the bones out of the oven. They should be browned and roasted.

Place the roasted bones in a large stockpot with a sieve, and fill the pot with water, covering the bones. Put more onion and garlic, the fennel (or anise), and the remaining herbs and spices in the pot and bring it to a boil.

Once boiling, reduce the heat to a simmer and leave to cook for 24 hours. This allows all the ingredients to mix together to create an amazing broth. When done, this recipe makes a wonderful broth for soups, gravies, stews, and whatever else you wish to use it for.

I have not bought an over-the-counter broth for over 10 years now, since I started making my own. The proof is in the broth for your base for homemade soups and stews!

Preparation time: 60 minutes
Cooking time: 24 hours
Yield: 32 cups broth

Serving size: 1 cup
Calories per serving: 130

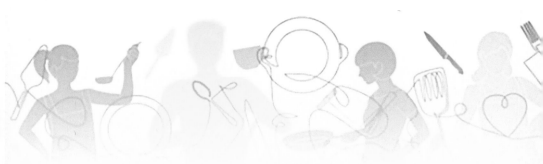

BISON SOUP

10 C broth
5 stalks celery, chopped
3 T Herbamare
2 onions, finely chopped
2 C wild rice
1 lb. ground bison
1 medium-sized fennel, finely chopped
1 clove garlic, chopped
½ lb. organic carrots, chopped
½ lb. frozen organic edamame
1/3 C house blend (optional)
salt to taste
pepper to taste
frozen peas

Note: Add the flour you desire a thicker soup. If you add cooked wild rice, you don't need to do so until later, right near the end, just prior to serving. If you add uncooked wild rice, then do so right at the beginning to allow it to cook all day. As wild rice takes over 45 minutes to an hour to cook on its own, within a soup it will take longer because it is cooking along with the other ingredients.

Place all ingredients in a large pot. Cover with the broth. Or if you use a slow cooker then principal is the same cover with broth. The only change is the slow cooker will take a minimum of 6 hours to cook thoroughly.

Use whatever meat you like. Brown meat in a pot first with olive oil, garlic, and onion until it has browned. add about 1/3 cup of flour to soak up the fat. Let the soup cook all day. Allowing all the flavors to marinate and mingle.

If you add other items to your soup such as lentils or beans, be sure to use more broth to accommodate these ingredients

Preparation time: 15 minutes
Cooking time: 1 hour to 6 depending on whether a slow cooker is used.

Yield: 15 cups
Serving size: 1.5 cups
Calories per serving: 21

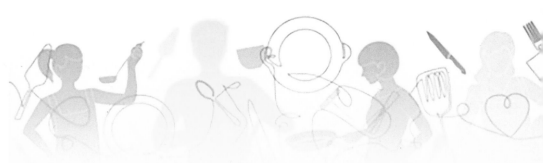

Chicken Soup

2 lbs. chicken (parts or leftover carcass from a roast chicken)
1 to 2 bay leaves
1 clove garlic, halved
1 medium-sized onion, quartered
½ t pepper
½ t poultry seasoning
½ t sage
½ t salt
¼ fresh fennel, quartered
water to cover

Place the roast chicken carcass or chicken parts in a large pot that will hold about 20 cups of water. A Dutch oven works well. Add all ingredients. Cover with water and bring to a boil. Turn the heat down and simmer for 2 hours. Once cooked, pull the bones and parts out to strain the broth. A clearer broth is achieved by skimming the film of fat off the top of the liquid as it is cooking. The broth can be further clarified by straining it through a strainer or cheesecloth. This broth can be stored and frozen either in jars or Ziplock bags or used for soup immediately.

Chicken soup is a simple meal. It is made by bringing to a boil and then simmering chicken parts and/or bones in water, with a variety of flavoring. The flavour of chicken is most potent when it is simmered in water with salt and only a few vegetables, such as onions, carrots, and celery. Variations on the flavour are gained by adding root vegetables such as parsnip, potatoes, sweet potatoes, and celery root; herbs such as parsley and dill; and other vegetables such as zucchini, whole garlic cloves, and tomatoes. Saffron or turmeric is sometimes added as a yellow colourant. Seasonings such as black pepper can be added too. The soup should be brought to a boil in a covered pot and cooked on a very low flame for 1 to 3 hours.

You can also use this recipe to make broth for turkey soup after you have cleaned the carcass from a turkey dinner. The nutritional value of chicken soup can be boosted by adding turkey meat to it, as turkey is a richer source of iron.

This broth to great for cooking and making soups, or for cooking wild rice.

Preparation time: 10 minutes
Cooking time: 2 hours
Yield: 15 cups

Serving size: 1.5 cups
Calories per serving: 185

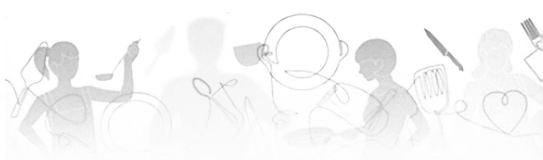

Pizza

3 C house blend
2 T olive oil
1¼ C buttermilk
1 T baking powder
1 egg white
1 T Coconut Sugar
1 T xanthan gum
¼ t garlic powder
¼ t oregano (or basil or Italian seasoning)
¼ t salt

Note: For buttermilk, I use almond milk left to sour for a few minutes with a teaspoon of lemon juice added. For additional suggestions, please see the section titled "Thickeners, Binders, Substitutions, and Other Additions." Also, egg replacer and egg white are fine to use instead of a real egg. Please keep in mind, though, that egg replacer does contain cornstarch, so use caution if you have issues with corn.

Note: for Yeast risen crust substitute the baking powder with 2 T gluten free yeast and take a quarter cup of almond milk out and warm it before adding the yeast to activate it before adding your liquid to dry ingredients, also adding a pinch of coconut sugar will further activate the yeast as well.

Preheat oven to 400 degrees.

In a large bowl, blend all dry ingredients together. Next, mix all wet ingredients together, then blend wet and dry ingredients until the dough forms into a ball.

Divide the dough ball in half and place both portions onto two pans lined with parchment paper. Place another piece of parchment paper on top and use a rolling pin to roll the dough out flat. Once this is done, take the top layer of parchment paper off. Put the desired toppings on the pizza dough and place it in the oven to cook for 15 to 20 minutes.

Choose your toppings and cheese that bring you happiness in your favorite pizza.

Preparation time: 15 minutes
Cooking time: 25 minutes
Yield: 2 large pizza crusts

Serving size: 1/16 as each pizza yields approximately 8 pieces
Calories per serving: crust only is 98

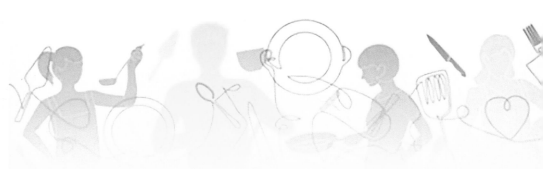

WILD RICE STUFFING

5 to 7 slices any gluten-free bread, chopped into small squares (your favorite bread)
3 T melted butter
2 C cooked wild rice
1 medium-sized yellow onion, finely chopped
½ t Himalayan sea Salt
¼ t Pepper
1 clove crushed garlic
poultry seasoning, fresh or dried
water to moisten

poultry seasoning made with about 3 tablespoons of a finely chopped combination of fresh rosemary and thyme.

Preheat oven to 350 degrees. Place the bread, wild rice, garlic and onion in a bowl. Mix the spices and poultry seasoning separately. Add the melted butter to the spice and seasoning mix and blend well. Then add this to the bread, wild rice, and onion combination and mix thoroughly. Moisten this mixture with water.

Take the mixture and stuff it into the bird until the cavity is full. If there is any leftover stuffing once this is done, you can put it into a foil bag and place it in the pan to cook with the bird in the oven. The rule of thumb when cooking a large bird is 13 minutes per pound, so if you have a 15-pound turkey, the total cooking time would be 3 hours and 25 minutes.

You can also choose not to stuff the turkey. In this case, place the stuffing in a pan to cook on its own 35 minutes prior to finishing preparing dinner. It will be ready in time for serving. We soak a turkey in a saltwater brine overnight and then cook then spatchcock the turkey to cook astewr and with a more even cooking. . I cook the stuffing separately, 30 minutes prior to serving dinner.

Preparation time: 20 minutes
Cooking time: varies depending on turkey

Yield: up to 8 servings
Serving size: ¾ cup
Calories per serving: 244

Teaching

I steam my vegetables. My family and I live in the Fraser Valley, where the vegetables are often reasonably priced when in season. Buying from local farmers means that you can purchase vegetables throughout the growing season at a fair price, and then buy organic at your regular grocery store during the off-season. This factors into what cooking and meal planning is all about. I often think about what meals to prepare days in advance. Figuring out what to feed my family is something I think about all the time, as my household is driven by food!

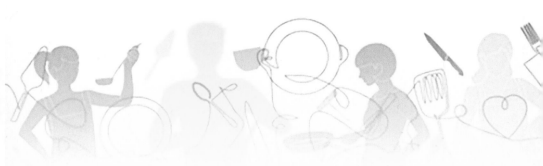

FRIED WILD RICE

3 stalks celery, finely chopped
2 shallots or 1 large-sized yellow onion, finely chopped
1 C cooked quinoa
4 - 6 T olive oil
2 T butter
1 t salt
2 T soya – we use Braggs Gluten free
2 T maple. Chokecherry or coconut syrups
½ C dried cranberries (optional)
½ t Himalayan sea salt
1/3 C chopped walnuts (optional)
½ cup pepitas – pumpkin seeds
¼ C cilantro, finely chopped
¼ of a medium sized fresh fennel, finely chopped
¼ t pepper
1 tsp turmeric
3 C wild rice
9-10 cups water

Put the wild rice, water, and salt in a large, heavy saucepan and bring it to a boil. Reduce this to a simmer and cook for 45 to 55 minutes, or until the rice seeds open up and the rice looks like it has completely "popped", and the inner whites are visible.

Put all the remaining ingredients in a large, heavy wok and sauté them until they are tender, and the flavours mingle. Then add the cooked wild rice and quinoa. Allow everything to mix. The ground turmeric gives this dish an antifungal boost. I use what works in my home and often I use what is available seasonally to work with. This is the favourite with my family and a ceremony feast must.

Preparation time: 15 minutes
Cooking time: 45 minutes for wild rice and 15 minutes additional time for frying

Yield: 15 servings
Serving size: 1.5 C
Calories:99

Story Time

When I first met Ken, we used to get together to eat in the lunchroom at work. He would bring his lunch bag . . . and it would have almost the same thing every day. Wild rice, meat, and veggies. There would be a huge amount of each. One day he came in to have lunch and had made this fried wild rice. It was delicious, so we started adding different things to it. Nowadays we add ground meat, diced-up chicken, stew meat, and whatever leftovers we have. It became a staple in our diets and remains so. He cannot eat them, but I like adding dried cranberries to it. if you can, try this dish with this option—you will love the little bit of sweetness it adds.

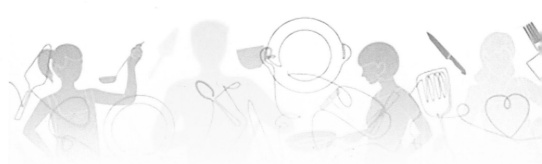

Mac 'n' Cheese

2 C uncooked gluten-free pasta
2 T house blend (heaping)
2 T margarine
1½ C almond milk or lactose free milk(unsweetened)
1½ C shredded cheese (your choice of cheese)

Note: total preparation time for this dish can be cut to 20 minutes. Gluten Free pasta cooks very quick – less than 6 minutes.

Melt the margarine in a medium-sized saucepan on the stove at a temperature of 6 to 7, or medium. Add the flour, stir until everything is blended. Use a whisk to ensure this mixture is creamy. Continuously stir it to make sure that there is no clumping. Add the almond milk gradually until it has fully blended. Add the shredded cheese and mix until it has melted and is well blended.

Place a large Dutch oven on the stove filled with about 6 cups of water, and bring it to a full, rolling boil. Add the pasta and reduce the heat to medium. Cook the pasta for about 6 to 8 minutes, until it is al dente. Drain the pasta and rinse it with cool water. Put the pasta back into the Dutch oven and pour the cheese sauce over it.

Preparation time: 5 minutes to boil water
Cooking time: 20 minutes for sauce
6 minutes for pasta
Yield: 4 servings
Serving size: 1½ cups
Calories per serving: 372

Teaching

Living gluten free requires reading everything and understanding what additives are in the foods you eat. It takes hours of research to determine whether there are additives that contain gluten or other items that may cause an allergic reaction. Not all gluten-free products are truly gluten free. The fewer ingredients there are, the more likely it is not to have a reaction. Watch out for "natural flavours"—they tend to be full of chemically altered facsimiles of a flavour, or additives such as organic material and fillers.

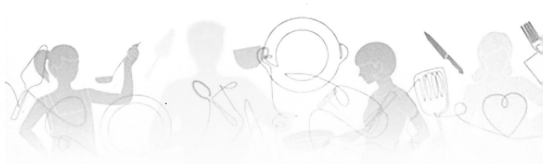

BANNOCK

3 C Signature blend
½ cup Psyllium
½ C Enriched Tapioca
3 T baking powder
4 t xanthan gum
1½-2 C warm water
2 eggs
1 t salt
¾ C lard

Preheat oven to 350 degrees. Line a cookie sheet with parchment paper.

Mix together the flour, baking powder, xanthan gum, and salt until well blended. Cut in lard until well blended. I have used Earth balance sticks for this recipe instead of lard.

Add warm water until the dough is sticky and forms into a moist ball. Remember that gluten-free dough needs to be moist and sticky to the touch. This is normal.

Take the dough and place on the cookie sheet, flattening it into round Bannock about 1 inch thick. Poke fork holes in it a few times.

Place the flattened dough in the oven for about 25 minutes. Remove and cool on a wire rack.

Preparation time: 10 minutes
Baking time: 25 minutes

Yield: 6 servings
Serving size: 1-piece 128g
Calories per serving: 342

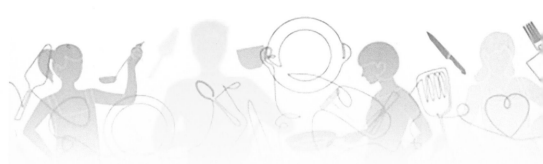

CHEDDAR BACON BISCUITS

1 T baking powder
4 T butter, cut into bits
3 C Signature blend
2 eggs or egg whites
1 C coconut Milk
1½ t xanthan gum
¼ t sea Salt
1 t coconut sugar
1 C aged Cheddar
1/3 C lactose free yoghurt
1/3 C lactose free sour cream
½ C oil
½ cup crumbled bacon (optional)

Preheat oven to 425 degrees. Grease a baking sheet or line one with parchment paper.

In a medium bowl, combine all dry ingredients and use a whisk to blend thoroughly. Add the wet ingredients and stir just until the dry ingredients are moistened.

Drop ¼-cup mounds of dough about 2 inches apart on the greased or parchment-lined baking sheet. Top the biscuits with extra cheese and bacon on top, Bake for about 10 to 12 minutes, or until golden brown.

Remove the biscuits from the oven and let them cool slightly. Serve them warm.

These biscuits are like the melt-in-your-mouth regular biscuits, but just a healthier, gluten-free version. They can be served with soy cheese unless you can tolerate regular cheese.

Preparation time: 10 minutes
Baking time: 10 to 12 minutes

Yield: 10 biscuits
Serving size: 135g
Calories per serving: 203

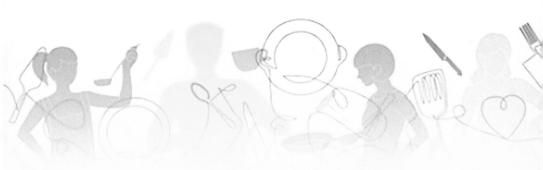

HAMBURGER AND HOTDOG BUNS

Dry Ingredients:

3 t sugar
2 C house blend
1 T psyllium
2 t xanthan gum
1 T baking powder
1 t salt
¼ C whey protein

Wet Ingredients:

1¼ C warm water
1 egg white
1 T yeast
¼ C oil (olive, coconut, etcetera)

Note: This recipe contains yeast.

Preheat oven to 350 degrees.

Mix all dry ingredients in a large bowl. Add the wet ingredients and stir to form a batter.

Line a baking pan with parchment paper. Drop the batter onto the parchment paper, leaving space for it to spread while baking. Once you add the wet ingredients, it is important to get this into the oven immediately. This is in order to benefit from the leavening process, which gives the buns their light and airy feel. Bake for about 20 to 25 minutes.

This versatile recipe is becoming a hamburger and sloppy joe mainstay in my home. It offers a great option for gluten-free eating.

Preparation time: 15 minutes
Baking time: 25 minutes

Yield: 6 buns
Serving size: 115g
Calories per serving: 152

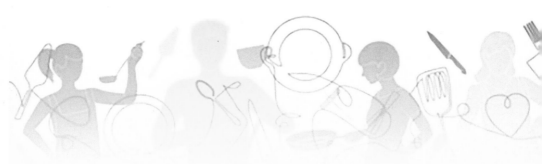

TORTILLAS

2 C Signature blend
2 T shortening
2 t xanthan gum
1½ t salt
1 t baking powder
1 t sugar
1 C warm water

Have a cast-iron flat pan or nonstick cooking pan on hand. A large, flat pan is preferable, as it is similar to a griddle. You can use a tortilla press to make the tortillas a uniform shape and thickness or use a good rolling pin to achieve thickness desired.

Turn on the heat to between 6 and 7, or almost to the maximum temperature, to ensure that the pan gets hot.

In a large bowl, add all dry ingredients and cut in the shortening. Add the warm water slowly until the dough becomes smooth.

Form the dough into balls roughly the size of tennis balls. Place the dough balls on a piece of parchment paper, and then place another piece of parchment on top. Roll the dough out until each ball is flat and circular. Each tortilla's thickness should be about ¼ inch for consistency. OR purchase a tortilla press from a local kitchen shop and us this with parchment to flatten your tortillas

Remove the top piece of parchment paper and turn the tortillas onto the hot pan. Heat each side of tortilla about 2 minutes per side to cook through.

Preparation time: 20 minutes
Cooking time: 30 minutes

Yield: 6 servings
Serving size: 125g
Calories per serving: 170

Historical Points of Interest

The stories of food are throughout my family and through historical research I found my Great great grandfather Chief August Jack Khahtsahano's journals written from 1932-1955 when they were published by Major John Matthews, my grandfathers' journals and the introduction of new foods carried interesting interactions. The introduction of molasses to the Khahtsahlano people, Chief August Jack conveyed this story to Major J. S. Matthews:

> "Then Whiteman's on schooner give molasses . . . Indian not know what it for, so Indian rub on leg (thighs and calves) for medicine. You know Indian sit on legs for long time in canoe; legs get stiff. Rub molasses on legs make stiffness not so bad. Molasses stick legs bottom of canoe. Molasses not much good for stiff legs, but my ancestors think so. Not their fault, just mistake; they do not know molasses well to eat." And then August Khatsahlano laughed heartily.

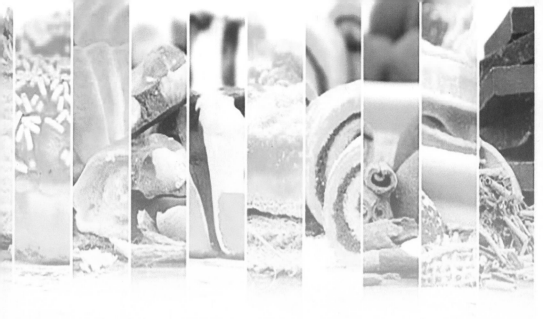

Sweet

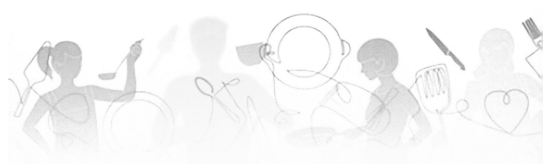

PANCAKES

2 C house blend
2 egg whites
2 t olive oil
1½ C almond milk or Lactose free milk
1½ t baking powder
¼ t salt
1 t Cinnamon

Note: If you prefer sugar in your mix, add a tablespoon to it prior to blending.

Blend all ingredients together with a stick blender in a large measuring cup. (I suggest using a 10-cup measuring cup in order to pour your batter onto the griddle as you cook the pancakes.)

Place the griddle on the burners. Use one of those large griddles that covers two burners on the stove. Make sure it is either nonstick or cast iron. Turn the burners on to just around medium too high to bring the temperature up to hot on the griddle. Put some olive oil on the griddle. When the pancakes are bubbling on top, flip them over for about 2 to 3 minutes per side. They will not be really brown because gluten-free pancakes do not brown the same as regular pancakes. They will, however, be fluffy and sugar free.

Variations: Add a mashed banana or ½ C chocolate chips. You can add 1 C Fresh or frozen blueberries as well.

Serve these pancakes with my strawberry sauce. Next recipe…

Preparation time: 10 minutes
Cooking time: 15 minutes

Yield: 12 to 15 medium-sized pancakes
Serving size: 119g
Calories per serving: 123

Story Time

I call these "roadhouse pancakes." Ken was on a road trip with Riel to Manitoba and texted me saying he needed a recipe for pancakes. I had nothing, so I jumped online immediately, piecing together recipes while making them in the kitchen as I texted him the ingredients! We fine-tuned our recipe to come up with these wonderful sugar-free pancakes. In fact, the picture here is one that Ken texted me from his cousin's house in Fisher Branch, Manitoba. This is also where Ken learned that altitude and air pressure made a huge difference in the amount of liquid and cooking temperature affected cooking. There was a need to change the liquid he used in making his pancakes for every province he travelled through. We developed the recipe while he was in Alberta, and he went from there to Saskatchewan and Manitoba. It was a lesson in science and experimentation for both of us.

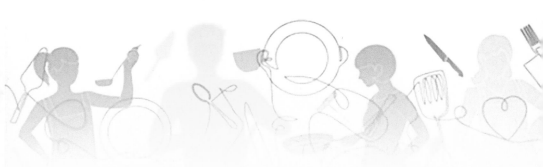

STRAWBERRY SAUCE

½ bag frozen strawberries (approximately 1 kg)
¼ C sugar, maple syrup or honey
4 t tapioca crystals
Juice of ½ lemon

Note: Try using whatever fresh fruit is in season and adjust the tapioca crystals to thicken!

Place all ingredients in a large Dutch oven on the stove.

Adjust the temperature to medium heat. Bring the fruit to a boil, and then lower the temperature to a simmer once the fruit heats up. Stir and let the fruit break down. I use a potato masher sometimes to help the fruit reduce completely.

This makes a rich sauce that is very yummy served with my pancakes. If the berries are started just before making the pancakes, everything should be ready at the same time.

Note: sweetener is optional only to add additional flavor to fruit – fresh fruit is sweeter

Preparation time: 5 minutes
Cooking time: 25 minutes for frozen fruit

15 minutes for fresh fruit

Yield:4 cups

Serving size: ¼ cup per 2 pancakes

Calories per serving: 16.5 and note if you use no stevia then the calorie count will decrease.

Thoughts

Sugar is not required in all foods—we fool ourselves into thinking we need to have sugar in everything we eat because we have grown up with a taste for it. Whipped cream, for example, does not require sugar; we add sugar just to make it sweeter. When we start eating food without sugar, we realize we don't need it. Fresh fruit are a perfect with their natural sugars. When I cook fruit, their own sugars often provide enough flavor.

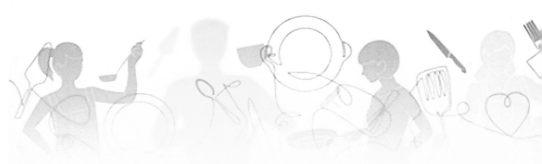

SQUAMISH BARS

This recipe is an altered version of Nanaimo bars and very delicious. This is a no bake recipe and uses only a food processor blender to make this. 9 x 9-inch bar pan

Base:

1.5 C unsweetened coconut
1.5 C Hazelnut or Almond flour*
½ C Coconut Oil melted
¾ C Coconut Sugar (Palm or organic)
¼ C Cocoa or raw cocoa powder
10 dates pitted
2 pinches of sea salt

Filling:

2 C or 2 packages Coconut Cream (*this product comes in a brick form and is just dried coconut meat)
½ C water
½ C maple syrup or coconut nectar
2 tsp Vanilla powder or Vanilla extract **
½ C Melted Coconut Oil
pinch of sea salt

Chocolate Ganache topping:

½ C Maple syrup
½ C Coconut oil
½ C Cocoa powder
1 tsp Vanilla Powder or Vanilla Extract

Filling

The filling can be done first by placing the ingredients into a bowl. I use a home proofer to help warm ingredients to blend or use a blender to mix. Pour on base and set in fridge to chill – 1 hour.

Base

In food processor grind the nuts finely, then add all ingredients for the crust together. Blend in food processor until a paste like consistency about 20 seconds and up to one minute. scrape the ingredients into the 9 x 9-inch bar pan and place in fridge for about an hour or freezer for about 10 minutes

Top

Take all ingredients for Chocolate topping and put in small blender. Blend ingredients until a smooth chocolate mixture is about 20 seconds. Spread the contents on top of the middle layer until evenly distributed. Chill in fridge for about 10-15 minutes or until top layer is firm. Use a bar cutter to cut. This freezes well. served chilled.

Preparation time: 45 minutes
Refrigeration time: 2- 3 hours
Yield: 30 squares
Calories per serving:224

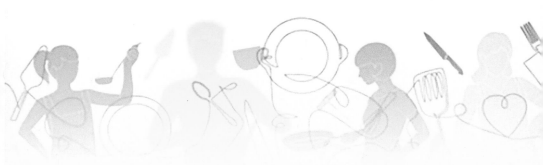

COFFEE CAKE

Cake:

3 C Signature blend
3 t xanthan gum
2 t baking powder
2 egg whites
2 t organic vanilla extract
1½ C buttermilk
1¼ C softened butter (20 T equivalent)
1 t baking soda
1 t salt
1 C Coconut sugar

Topping:

1 T cinnamon
¾ C nuts (your choice; I used walnuts)
½ C coconut sugar

Preheat oven to 350 degrees. Line a 13" x 9" x 2" baking pan with parchment paper.

Mix all dry ingredients together in a large bowl. Add softened butter and mix until crumbly. Remove 1 cup of mixture and set aside.

Mix all wet ingredients together. Add wet ingredients to the dry and mix well, until a smooth batter forms. Pour the mixture into the parchment-lined baking dish.

Mix the topping ingredients together in a small bowl and add the reserved 1-cup crumb mixture to this. Sprinkle it on top of the cake evenly and place in the oven to bake for about 50 to 60 minutes, or until toothpick comes out clean.

Preparation time: 20 minutes
Baking time: 50 to 60 minutes

Yield: 12 servings
Serving size: 147g
Calories per serving: 469

Story Time

Ken and Riel are always bugging me for sweets. They wanted coffee cake they could eat, and it was a challenge to come up with the perfect recipe! Do you know just how hard it is to find a coffee cake that is gluten free and almost sugar free? Well, here it is! This coffee cake is pretty good, if I say so myself!

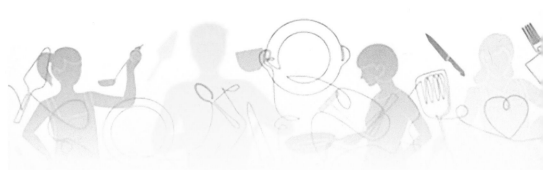

CINNAMON BUNS

Part 1:

3 C house blend
½ C Psyllium
2 packages quick-rise yeast
¾ C coconut sugar
¾ C softened butter
¼ C xanthan gum

Part 2:

6 eggs (or egg whites)
6 to 10 C flour (depending on need)
water to make 3 cups liquid (lukewarm)

Filling:

3 T cinnamon
2 to 3 C coconut sugar
1¼ C butter

Icing:

4 T cream cheese
3 C icing sugar

2 T butter
1 t organic vanilla extract

Preheat oven to 350 degrees. Line two 13" x 9" x 2" pans with parchment paper.

Mix together all ingredients in part one and blend well. Set aside. Mix together all ingredients in part two. Add this to part one, and then add flour as required until the mixture forms a wet, sticky dough. It should form a dough that is tacky and can be rolled out onto parchment paper to about a ¾-inch thickness. You will need a large surface area for rolling out this dough. I suggest working on a large counter.

Knead the dough and place it in a bowl to rise for about 1 to 1½ hours. It should double in size. Melt the butter and add the coconut sugar and cinnamon to it. Take the dough and place it on a floured surface. Roll it out to about a ¾-inch thickness. You can also use parchment paper to ease the rolling. Pour the butter, coconut sugar, and cinnamon filling mixture onto the dough surface and spread it around with a spatula until the dough is evenly covered—this is sticky business!

Start carefully rolling the dough at one end until the buns are completely rolled into a large log. Cut into the log to create buns about 1½ inches thick, and then place them in the parchment-lined pans about a ½ inch apart to give them space to expand. Allow the buns to rise for about 30 minutes. Bake them for about 30 to 45 minutes. This is a good time to combine all ingredients for the icing. When the buns have doubled in size and browned, they are ready. Remove them from the oven and allow them to cool for about 10 minutes. Put the icing on top. They can also be enjoyed without it.

Preparation time: 30 minutes
Resting time: 30 minutes for first rising
                30 minutes for second rising
Baking time: 25 minutes
Yield: 18 buns
Serving size: 337g
Calories per serving: 715

Story Time

These cinnamon buns are a creation I came up with years ago when commercial cinnamon bun shops first arrived on the scene. I craved these ooey, gooey delights, so I fiddled around with a sweet bread recipe until I got the right mixture using regular flour. Back then, my original filling mixture contained demerara sugar, butter, good-quality cinnamon, and sometimes raisins. These ingredients made for heavenly cinnamon buns! Today, I have revamped my original recipe to make it gluten free, using coconut sugar instead, and it has turned out really well with my house blend flour. Friends and family beg me for this recipe whenever I make a batch of buns!

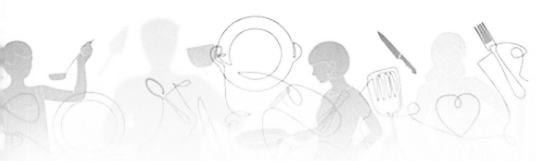

Banana Bread

4 egg whites
4 C Signature blend flour
3 t xanthan gum
2½ t baking soda
2 t cinnamon
2 t organic vanilla extract
1¾ C mashed bananas (3 to 5 large and overripe)
1 C coconut sugar
1 t salt
¾ C buttermilk
¾ C softened butter

Note: Fresh or frozen bananas work fine for this recipe. And egg replacer can be used in lieu of real egg whites—just follow the directions on the package. I have also used applesauce or chia seeds, excellent substitutes for egg whites or egg replacer too.

Preheat oven to 350 degrees. Line two loaf pans with parchment paper.

Mix the flour, baking soda, salt, and xanthan gum in a bowl and set aside.

Mix the coconut sugar and butter together, and then add the bananas, egg whites, and buttermilk. add in the cinnamon and vanilla extract and blend until creamy.

Add the dry ingredients to the wet and stir until well mixed.

Pour the batter into the loaf pans and bake in the oven until the loaves rise and are brown, about 55 to 60 minutes.

Cool the loaves for about 5 minutes. Pull them out of the pans and cool them fully prior to cutting them into slices.

This recipe originally also had maraschino cherries, chocolate chips, and walnuts. Feel free to add ¾ cup of each of those ingredients if you wish.

Preparation time: 20 minutes
Baking time: 55 to 60 minutes

Yield: 2 loaves, with about 8 pieces each
Serving size: 132g
Calories per serving: 197

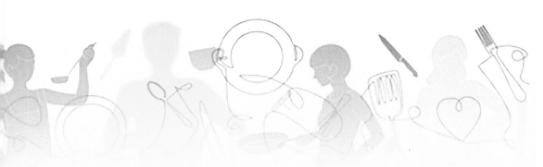

FRESH FRUIT PIE

3 C whole cranberries, fresh or frozen
2 pie crusts (see next recipe) or use ready made shells
½ C coconut sugar (or stevia)
¼ C tapioca crystals
pinch of salt

Note: Use whatever fruit you wish. It should be precooked to thicken it prior to filling the pie crust and baking.

Preheat oven to 350 degrees.

Put the fruit in a pot and mix in the tapioca and coconut sugar (or stevia) on low to medium heat. Watch this mixture closely until the fruit breaks down. As the fruit cooks it will thicken, so the temperature should be reduced to a low simmer and then shut off completely. This process takes about 30 minutes.

Roll out one of the pie crust pastries and place it in a pie plate. Take a ladle or large spoon and pour the fruit mixture into the pie crust, but do not overfill it.

Gently apply the second pie crust over the fruit filling. Use a fork to press down the edges of the top crust so that it seals together with the bottom crust. With a knife, pierce the top pie crust.

You can glaze the top crust with a beaten egg and sprinkle it with sugar if desired.

Place the pie in the oven and bake it for about 25 to 30 minutes, until the crust turns golden brown.

Preparation time: 20 minutes
Baking time: 30 minutes

Yield: 1 pie, with about 8 servings
Serving size: 55g
Calories per serving : 142

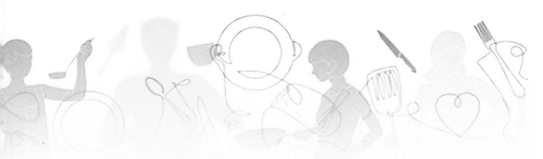

PIE CRUST

2¼ C + 1 T signature blend flour
2 T lemon juice
2 T water
1 t baking powder
1½ t xanthan gum
1 egg white
1 t salt
1 T stevia/coconut sugar
¾ C vegan lard or shortening

Note: I have used many different types of lards and fats, and I have found through trial and error that the best type is Earth Balance Shortening or the same brand's "butter sticks". This recipe has used lard, shortening and vegan butter sticks. The difference is in the absorption of the fat in the flour – each fat requires a slightly different amount of flour in blending, and this is done by feel in mixing the flour and fat together. Combine all dry ingredients. Add the lard or shortening and mix until well blended. The consistency should be as pea-like as possible.

Mix all wet ingredients. Add them to the dry ingredients and form a ball of dough.

I use parchment paper to roll out my pastry dough. I place the dough on the paper and put another piece of parchment paper on top of the dough. Then I roll out the dough to the appropriate size and thickness before placing it in the pie plate. This pastry dough is a little more fragile than the regular kind, but it is very flaky and delicious once baked.

Preparation time: 20 minutes
Yield: Four 9-inch crusts; 2 tops, 2 bottom
Serving size: 55g
Calories per serving: 14

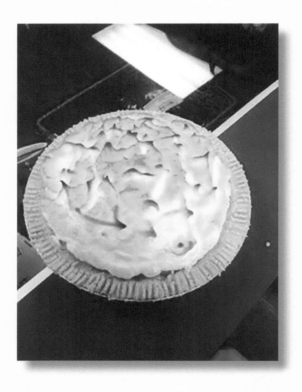

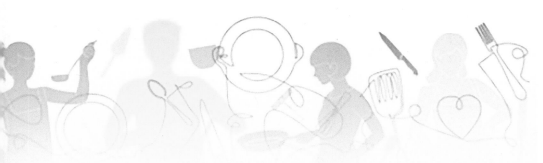

REGULAR HOMEMADE PIE CRUST

5 to 6 C flour (regular flour)
1 egg
1 lb lard (not shortening)
1 t salt
1 t vinegar
water

Crack the egg into a cup, add the vinegar, and then add enough water to make 1 cup. Mix with a fork vigorously. Set aside.

Pour the flour into a large bowl and add the salt. Cut in the lard. Mix in the lard until the flour feels clumpy. Once the lard is thoroughly blended with the flour, the mixture will have a crumbly, pea-like consistency. Add the egg, vinegar, and water mix. Blend this in with a spoon and then with your hands until a dough is formed. If needed, add more flour until the dough can be formed into a large ball. Knead the dough to make it elastic and even. You do not want it to be sticky, so use flour to make sure it is smooth and pliable.

This recipe will make enough dough for about four to five large pies.

Preparation time: 20 minutes

Yield: Ten 9-inch crusts; 5 tops, 5 bottom
Serving size: 184g
Calories per serving: 290

Story Time

This is the only non-gluten-free recipe in my book, but I included it because it has been the cornerstone of my life for as long as I can remember. It has also been the one thing my entire family still relies on me to bake for them. My granny, Eva, used to make pies and take them to sell at the Mosquito Creek Marina in North Vancouver every week. The money she raised helped feed her family. I asked my mom how to make pies when I was about five years old. She laughed but described the ingredients and the process. I came back from the kitchen a couple of hours later and showed her what I had made. Mom was so impressed she was speechless! this is a beloved family tradition passed down from dear Granny Eva.

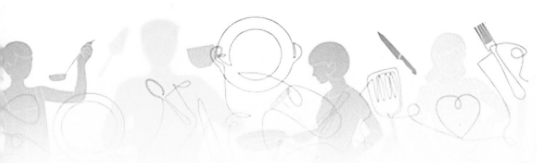

ALMOND COCONUT TART

Pastry:

Use Pie Crust recipe

Filling:

3 egg whites
2 C unsweetened desiccated coconut
1½ C honey
1 C ground almonds
½ C house blend
¼ C coconut oil
¼ t salt

Preheat oven to 350 degrees. Roll out the pie crust onto the bottom of a 13" x 9" x 2" pan.

Mix the filling and pour half of it into the pie crust. Put 2/3 of the crumble topping on the syrup.

Place the tart into the oven for 25 minutes, or until it is golden brown.

Take any remaining pie crust and divide it into balls. Wrap them in parchment paper and freeze them until a later time. Take any of the remaining crumble topping and freeze it as well.

Preparation time: 30 minutes
Baking time: 25 minutes

Yield: 15 bars
Serving size: 150g
Calories per serving: 549

<u>Teaching</u>
Cooking and baking are similar to science—experimentation is necessary in order to find what works. The majority of my recipes are old recipes collected over years, handed down from family and sometimes parts of recipes scrounged through old cookbooks in my collection. It is necessary to make adjustments to get the right texture, get the desired taste, and meet the appropriate needs when entering the world of gluten free. We all commonly adjust spices to taste, so recipes with flours are no different. They too require trial and error to achieve success.

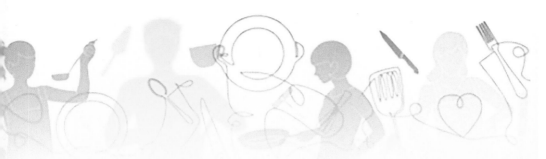

Carrot Cake with Cream Cheese Icing

Cake:
Dry indgredients

2 t baking powder
2 t cinnamon
¾ t salt
2 C signature blend
2 t xanthan gum
1½ C Coconut sugar
1 t baking soda
½ C chopped nuts
½ t nutmeg

Wet ingredients:

2 C grated carrots
1 C drained crushed pineapple
3 egg whites
1 t organic vanilla extract
¾ C olive oil

Icing:

8 oz cream cheese – lactose free
3 C icing sugar
1 t organic vanilla extract

Note: You can use whatever oil and nuts you prefer. I use olive oil and walnuts.

Preheat oven to 350 degrees. Grease and flour a 13" x 9" x 2" pan or line it with parchment paper.

In a large bowl, mix together all dry ingredients. In a separate large measuring cup, mix together all wet ingredients. Stir the wet ingredients into the dry ingredients together only until blended.do not over stir.

Spread this mixture evenly into your greased or parchment-lined pan. Place it into the oven for about 40 minutes, until the center of the cake is evenly brown, or a toothpick comes out clean. Let the cake cool in the pan on a rack before icing and cutting it into squares.

If you would like to serve this cake with cream cheese icing, simply blend the icing ingredients until creamy and spread on top of the cake once it is cool.

Preparation time: 20 minutes
Baking time: 40 minutes

Yield: 12 servings
Serving size: 181g
Calories per serving: 435

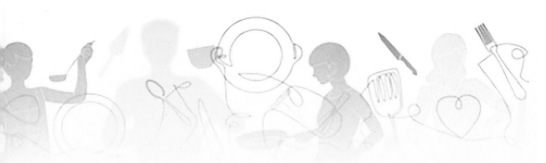

ALL-OCCASION CAKE

Vanilla Cake:

5 egg whites
2 t baking powder
½ tsp baking soda
1 tsp salt
2 C signature blend
2 t xanthan gum
1 C almond milk or lactose free milk
1 T organic vanilla extract
½ C softened butter
1¼ C coconut sugar or cane sugar
pinch of salt

Chocolate cake:

Add ¾ Cup unprocessed cocao and remove ½ cup of flour to adjust for cocao.

topping

2 cups fresh heavy whipping cream
Fresh fruit – about 2 cups for decoration

Note: You can also use blueberries or raspberries instead of strawberries.

Preheat oven to 350 degrees. Line a 13" x 9" x 2" pan with parchment paper.

In a large mixing bowl, mix together all wet ingredients and the stevia. In a separate measuring cup, mix together all dry ingredients. Blend the dry ingredients in with the wet and mix with an electric mixer for 2 minutes, scraping the sides of the bowl to ensure proper blending. Scrape the batter into the parchment-lined pan and spread it evenly. Place the pan in the oven and bake for 20 to 25 minutes. The cake will turn slightly brown. Remember that gluten-free baked items do not always turn completely brown when ready. it is important to watch the cake closely. It will be done when it bounces to the touch and a toothpick inserted comes out clean.

Remove the cake from the oven. Allow it to cool in the pan on a rack for 10 minutes before turning it out onto the rack to cool completely and removing the parchment paper.

Decorate the cake with fresh whipped cream and fruit just prior to serving.

Variation: upside down cake – use fruit (frozen or fresh 3-4 cups with 2 t blsp tapioca crystals sprinkled on fruit in large 10x13 baking dish. Pour half the cake mix over the fruit and bake. The remaining cake batter can be used for cupcakes.

Preparation time: 20 minutes
Baking time: 25 minutes
Decorating time: 20 minutes
Yield: 10 servings
Serving size: 175g
Calories per serving: 433

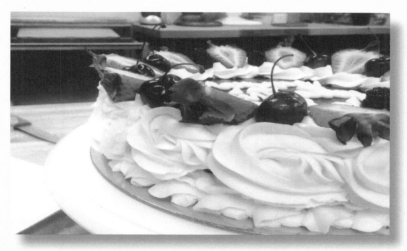

Variations on the cakes by using icing and fruit for decorations. I used a butter cream icing for this cake in my bakery YBGF in Mission.

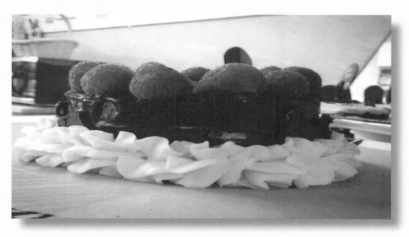

This tarlette was covered in our chocolate ganache made from maple syrup and unprocessed cacao

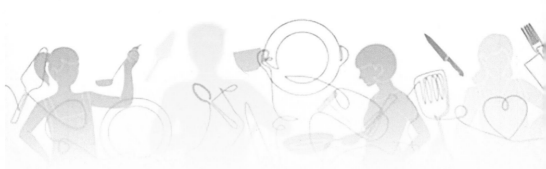

Avacado Chocolate Mousse Cake

Use Chocolate cake recipe or I also like to use the XO Baking Company chocolate cake mix for a quicker recipe.

Chocolate Cake
5 egg whites
2 t baking powder
½ tsp baking soda
1 tsp salt
1 1/2 C signature blend
¾ Cup unprocessed dark cacao
2 t xanthan gum
1 C almond milk or lactose free milk
1 T organic vanilla extract
½ C softened butter
1¼ C coconut sugar or cane sugar
pinch of salt

Preheat oven to 350 degrees

Blend cake mix and bake in parchment lined spring form pan to create a round cake. Bake for 30 minutes until center bounces back to touch or tooth pick is clean. Remove Cake to cool completely.

Avacado Mousse:
4-5 ripe Avacados
¾ cup maple syrup
¾ cup unprocessed unsweetened cacao

Clean avacados out of the shells and into a blender. Add maple syrup and cacao and blend until creamy and smooth. Pour this onto the cooled cake and decorate with fresh fruit.

Story Time
This cake became the favorite of Ken and our family for cakes. the combination of chocolate cake with the avocado mousse which is silky and smooth once chilled . You cannot tell there is avocados, and this cake is decadent and healthy...I made this cake in our Bakery and it became a special-order cake for many...

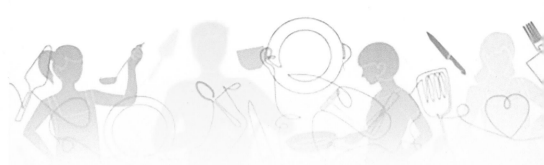

ANGEL FOOD CAKE

140g   (2 C)   Signature Flour
¾ cup coconut sugar
1 tsp salt
1 ¾ cup egg whites (approximately 10-12 eggs)
¼ C warm water
1 ½ tsp cream of tartar
1 tsp vanilla
1 tsp orange zest or almond extract
¾ C + 2 tbsp Coconut sugar (powdered in blender)

Directions:

Pre heat Oven to 350 degrees

Sift powder sugar and flour together add salt and sift 2-3 times to make light and fluffy.

In mixer whip egg whites to soft peask, add flour in 3-4 times carefully to blend flour and egg whites.

Pour cake mix into angel food cake pan bake in over for 25-30 minutes. Cake will be spongy to touch when fully baked.

If pouring cake batter onto parchment lined sheet pan then bake 10-12 minutes.

Cool thoroughly before removing from pan.

Layered sponge cake :

Using sheet pan for cake cut the cooled baked cake into three sections. On the first layer whip cream and fruit place a layer of cake on the fruit and repeat whip cream and fruit add third layer of cake and top with whip cream and fruit.

Angel food cake :

Cut cake and add fruit and whip cream and serve

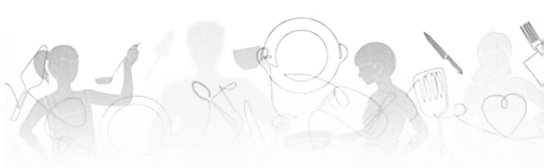

DATE SQUARES

Filling:

2 ½ cups whole pitted dates
1 ½ Cup water

Put this on stove in medium sized pot to simmer for about 10 minutes. (they should be soft and stewed to a mash like substance)

Crumb and Base topping:

1 ½ Cup Oats
1 ½ Cups Quinoa Flakes
1 Cup Almond Flour
¼ Cup Coconut Sugar
½ tsp Cinnamon
½ tsp salt
½ cup almond butter (or nut butter of your choice)
½ cup maple syrup
¼ cup melted coconut oil (butter or margarine is great too)

Preheat oven to 350 degrees. Lightly grease and line a 9 inch square pan with parchment paper. Blend the crumb dry ingredients together.

In a small glass bowl put maple syrup and nut butter and coconut oil together and heat slightly in microwave to blend better. Add to crumb ingredients and mix thoroughly.

Press half the crumb into the bottom of the square pan.

Spread the warm date filling on the base.

Drop the crumble remaining on the top and place in oven for 28-30 minutes.

Remove from oven and allow to cool before cutting.

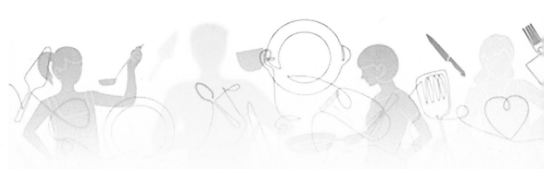

LEMON SQUARES

Base:

1 Cup Signature Blend Flour
1 tsp Xanthan Gum
½ cup butter
1/8 tsp salt

Top:

¾ Cup Cane sugar
¾ Cup unsweetened shredded coconut
3 eggs
3 Tbsp Honey
Juice and rind of one lemon

Preheat oven to 350 degrees, place parchment paper in an 8x 8 square pan.

Blend base and press into the square pan.

Mix the topping together and pour onto the base. Place in oven and bake for 35-40 minutes.

Allow to cool thoroughly before cutting

Story Time

The recipes I have gathered over the years have been from all walks in my life. I have family on my dads sides who taught me so much about food and to love and appreciate food from all walks of life

My friend Arlene is one of my wonderul inspirational friends. I used her lemon square recipe for its beautiful simplicity and use of fresh lemon. Arlene taught me how to bake and cook and make wonderul handmade soap...a story for another book...

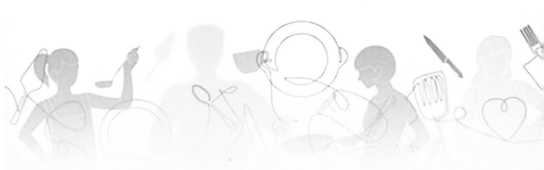

COCONUT POWER BARS

2 C coconut chips (150 g)
2 C unsweetened desiccated coconut (150 g)
2 egg whites
1 to 1½ C pumpkin seeds
1 C chopped almonds
¾ C coconut oil
¾ C honey (coconut sugar or maple syrup)
¾ C signature blend

Note: If you are not allergic to dried fruit, you can add 1 cup of raisins, dried cranberries, dried blueberries, etcetera to your liking to change up this recipe.

Preheat oven to 350 degrees. Put the coconut oil and sugar or honey or maple syrup in a saucepan and heat until the butter is melted. Take off the heat and leave to cook slightly.

Place flour into a mixing bowl and add all the remaining ingredients. Stir with a wooden spoon until everything is well blended. Tip the mixture into a prepared tin or pan and press down using the back of a spoon.

Bake in the oven for 20 to 25 minutes, until the top is golden brown, and the mixture feels firm to the touch.

Let the mixture cool completely in the tin or pan. Then transfer it onto a chopping board and cut it into bars. These bars keep for up to five days if stored in an airtight container.

Preparation time: 10 minutes
Baking time: 25 minutes

Yield: about 12 bars
Serving size:132g
Calories per serving: 466

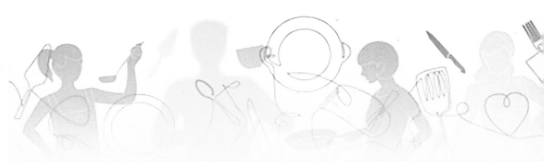

OAT BARS

1 Cup Butter or margarine
2 Cups coconut sugar
3 1.2 Cup Oats
2 tsp Baking powder
¼ tsp salt

Preheat oven to 350 degrees

Combine butter, sugar in sauce pany, when melted, set aside. Blend oats, salt and baking powder, add the melted butter and sugar.

Blend thoroughly and pour onto parchment lined cookie sheet.

The mixture can be flattened onto the cookie sheet with a piece or parchment on top and use a rolling pin to roll the surface of the bars flat and even distributed over the pan.

Bake for 25 minutes the bar should look like a molten mass of sugary oats.

Let cool completely before cutting.

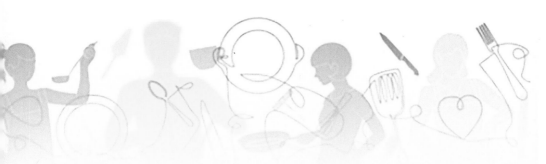

FIDDLE DIDDLES

Syrup:

2 ½ Cups or 350g Coconut Sugar
½ tsp Vanilla
¾ Cup or 105g unprocessed cacao
¾ Cup coconut Milk

Dry Ingredients:

1¾ Cup Quinoa Flakes or Oats (your choice)
1 ¼ Cup unsweetened shredded Coconut
1 ¼ Cup Puffed quinoa cereal

Directions place the syrup ingredients into a pot on the stove on low to medium heat, stir and cook until it comes to a rolling boil and take off stove immediiately. Set aside.

Mix all dry ingredients together and pour hot syrup over this misture and stir to blend well. Use an icecream scoop or measure scoop for cookies to scoop the mixture onto a parchment lined sheet. They will form chocolate balls you can place close togher on sheet. Once you fill the sheet place in freezer to set for about an hour.

These are so popular with my kids and husband that I had to make these by the hundreds.

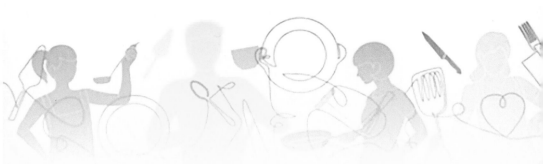

DATE ALMOND COOKIES

Makes about 20

Ingredients:

Filling:

12 oz. Pitted Dates
4 Tbsp Unsweetened Apple Sauce
2 Tbsp Honey or maple syrup
Pinch of cinnamon

Dough ingredients:

3 Cups almond flour (with husks for a darker colour)
½ tsp salt
¾ Cup maple syrup or honey
¼ Cup grapeseed or olive oil
1 Tbsp Vanilla

Directions:

Preheat oven to 350 degrees

Place parchment on a large cookie sheet pan.

Place filling into a blender and mix until forms a paste

Place dough ingredients into a meduium size mixing bowl, combine until well blended and a sticky dough forms. Place the dpough in a saran wrap and put in fridge to chill for one hour.

Divide the doung into four equal parts and roll between parchment paper to form a flat sheet with the dough about ¼ inch thick. Spread ¼ of the date filling on half the almond sheet, fold olver using parchment paper and place on sheet pan to bake. Repeat this until all four pieces are ready to bake. Bake for about 10-12 minuted, the almond dough should start to brown at the endges.

Remove and place on cooling racks until fully cooled before cutting. These are like a fig newton replacement – but much better!.

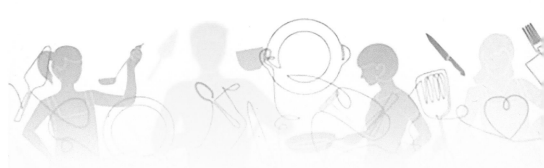

GINGER MOLASSES COOKIES

Ingredients:

2 ¾ Cup Signature blend flour
1 ¼ tsp Xanthan gum
2 ½ tsp baking soda
1 ¼ Cup Brown Sugar
1 Cup Margarine or Butter
2 free range eggs
1 ¼ tsp Cinnamon
¾ tsp cloves
¾ tsp ginger
½ Cup molasses

Directions:

Preheat oven to 350 degrees

Prepare a cookie sheet with parchment

Mix all ingredients in a mixing bowl using your dough hook (unless your really strong and can mix with a wooden spoon). Scoop with a cookie ball scoop and place on sheet pan about 2 inches apart. Bake for

8-10 minutes. Let cool on sheet before transfer to cool rack. Gluten free cookies are really soft when hot out of oven and need to cool before they can be handled.

Plants and herbs

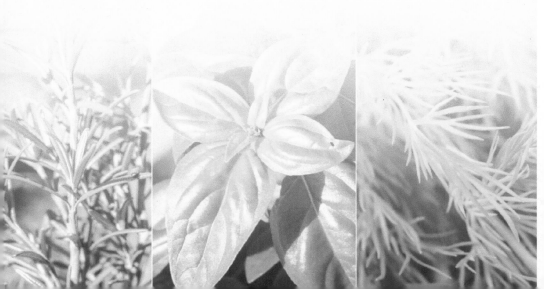

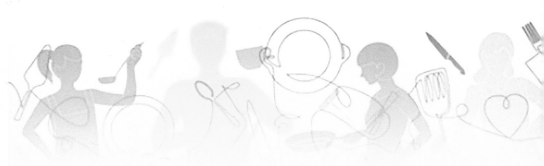

Herbals, plants, fungus and Tea

My own knowledge of teas is from spending time with my sister Dr. Cease Wyss and her daughter who own the Raven and Hummingbird Tea Co. I have also spent over a decade harvesting and working with elders here in Cree territory. I will share a few of the teas, plants and fungus I have harvested and some of their uses within our home. The sharing of these plants is to encourage you to explore these more. The written knowledge here of these is only for sharing personal experiences with these plants purposes and not meant to be educational.

Dandelion

Tea made from this common weed is mildly diuretic. Some women use it to reduce premenstrual bloating. Harvested in spring and used also in salves for burns, skin rash and eczema. Last year's harvest was made into a salve first placing the dandelions in oil for over 8 weeks and then blending with beeswax and coconut oil to create a salve.

Elderberry

Extracts of elder are sometimes used in over-the-counter cold remedies, and elderberry tea may alleviate cold and flu symptoms. Elderflowers and ripe elderberries are safe, but avoid the roots, stems, and leaves.

The tea is also a mild stimulant. I planted the black elder berry bushes in our home and had our first harvest of berries in the third summer of growth.

Chaga

A mushroom family growth on old birch. We have harvested this all over Alberta north of Red Deer. The small burnt looking growth are a fungus, and many teachings say to use this for women's hot flashes (personally it works!). it is used for tumor reduction and cancer support immune supports.

Labrador

Still found in bogs, the Labrador plant's aromatic young twigs, leaves, and flowers have long been used both fresh and dried for tea. It is a good medicine for colds and sore, irritated throats. The tea should be weak; a small handful of leaves steeped in boiling water for five minutes yields a pleasant beverage.

Nettle

Made from the same plant that causes stinging skin irritation, nettle tea is rich in vitamin C and several minerals. Herbalists recommend it to treat arthritis and gout, and to increase milk production in nursing mothers. It is good for steaming sinus's and drinking as tea for sinus infections.

Peppermint

Tea from this mint plant is refreshing and may stimulate digestion. It should, however, be avoided by anyone with a hiatal hernia, because peppermint promotes reflux of the stomach contents into the esophagus. Domestic growth of mint is easy, and I have several varieties in my annual gardens.

Wild Mint

Wild mint is found harvested near swamp and water ways along the banks, it hides among long grasses. Wild mint is used in ceremonies for tea. We harvest the mint in summer and use tea at home for health.

Raspberry Leaf

Herbalists recommend raspberry leaf tea to ease menstrual cramps. A plant and fruit that west coast women have used for centuries for treating women health. The shoots in early spring are loaded with vitamins and are tender and can be eaten picked fresh. The leaves and fruit can be used fresh or dried for teas.

Rose Hip

Rich in vitamin C, rose hip tea can substitute as an alternative to orange juice. I harvest these in fall late when frost is close, and they are abundant and dry on the bushes.

Story Time

My family and I go to North Vancouver to the Harmony Garden, a community garden built in the heart of the Capilano Reserve on Squamish Nation land. It is the brainchild of Elders, my mother and Dad among them. They approached the band and asked for permission to use a deserted piece of land that people were utilizing as a garbage dump. Soon this area was transformed into a thriving community garden to support the community kitchen my mother and sister created at St. Paul's Church in North Vancouver to feed people with little or no access to good, nutritional food. This kitchen has been in operation for over twenty years now, and the community garden is in its 20th year. My sister has been the champion and main source of work for this garden after our dad passed. Harmony Garden provides many of the fresh vegetables and herbs used by the community kitchen, as well as indigenous medicines and berries. My children have worked in the garden in the summertime, earning a little cash and gaining a lot of experience. We are always guaranteed a pot of tea made with fresh picks from the garden my sister has put together, including berries, herbs, and natural medicines. These experiences are always a wonderful treat.

AUTHORS FINAL NOTES

In closing I leave a few thoughts for people. The journey to change the way you eat is a personal one. Everyones health needs and food choices are their own. The journey for us was one that took us through history research – looking at our family history and indigneous peopls history to look at food and health. These are some ways in which we came to create a diet that worked for our family. To us food is central to everything we do. The way we feel after we eat is a large part of all celebrations and all things we do daily.

Approaching food from more than a nutritional base was important to us. The removal of processed food was a large part of changing our diet and our childrens approach to life as well. The change has improved our childrens growth, health and knowledge to make choices for themselves. I love when I talk to my adult children now and ask them what they wish to eat – most of the time its what can we make at home, or now we do tail gate picnics at grocery stores on the road instead of fast food restaurants.

When I research food I use the big research engines like google to look for information on flours I want to use and things I do not know about. When we started to use gluten free flours It was hours of reading and seeking out how best to cook and bake with these things. My book offers some of the best recipes we "trial and errored" with a bit of success. When I research I tend to seek out several sites for research and only chose what appealed to me having simple information and providing access to additional research.

I share some of our stories in the little boxes to break up the fact this is a cookbook. The journey for us was a bit of story telling and a bit of adventure to find the right path. We have been on this journey now for over 10 years. The things we learned in how to eat better, came with many stories. The wild rice was an entire journey – learning how vital this food was to trade, sustenance and ceremony. We learned that wild rice is a grass and harvested on lakes shores that are marshy and its a sustainable food that has been here for centuries. These stories made our journey so much fun. Our wild rice has come from athabasca Alberta, Hudson Bay Manitoba and Cranberry Portage Manitoba.

Our children and us made a little business of teaching and selling wild rice at pow wows, gatherings of our ceremony family and used for trade and donation to community gatherings with our bringing this only to ceremony. Our family knows us for our wild rice and that is one food we made time to learn about. We hope you take away the gift we recevied in learning abut using love and joy to cook at home and put beautifil energy into making your meals and cooking for your family. The food tastes so much better when intention and love are put into the food. We are grateful for the beautiful life we have – the cree say "Kinanaskomowin Miyo Pimatisown". This book and all our recipes are made in our home with this in mind daily...

Pihew Piyisew Iskwew

Sti7hay Sla7nay

Yvonne Wyss

BIBLIOGRAPHY

Davis, William. *Wheat Belly: Lose the Wheat, Lose the Weight, and Find Your Path Back to Health.* Emmaus, Pennsylvania: Rodale Press, 2011.

Junger, Alejandro. *Clean Gut: The Breakthrough Plan for Eliminating the Root Cause of Disease and Revolutionizing Your Health.* San Francisco: Harper One, 2013.

Matthews, James Skitt. *Early Vancouver* (vols. 1, 2). Vancouver: City of Vancouver, 2011.

Nahanee, Teressa Ann and Wyss, Barbara. *Inter-Tribal Cookbook: Recipes of North American Indians; Traditional and Modern.* Lone Butte, British Columbia: BRT Publishers, 1982.

Ustlahn Social Society. *Berry Cakes: Past and Present Diet of the Squamish People; A Story of Food and Cultural Change over 200 Years.* North Vancouver: Ustlahn Social Society, 2010.

Coconut oil: Benefits, uses, and controversy (medicalnewstoday.com) Used for research on coconut oils.

The 14 Best Gluten-Free Flours (healthline.com)

(picture of Ken and me)
Author Yvonne Bonnie Wyss
ywyss@mccedu.ca
2023

Ingram Content Group UK Ltd.
Milton Keynes UK
UKHW050244100623
423216UK00001B/2